Speaking Honestly with Sick
and Dying Children and Adolescents

Speaking Honestly with Sick and Dying Children and Adolescents

Unlocking the Silence

Dietrich Niethammer, M.D.

Foreword by Christoph Schmeling-Kludas, M.D.
Foreword by Ruprecht Nitschke, M.D.

Translated by Victoria W. Hill

The Johns Hopkins University Press
Baltimore

The Johns Hopkins University Press
2715 North Charles Street
Baltimore, Maryland 21218-4363
www.press.jhu.edu

Authorized translation of the first German-language edition of
D. Niethammer, *Das sprachlose Kind*, © 2008 by Schattauer
GmbH, Stuttgart/Germany

Library of Congress Cataloging-in-Publication Data
Niethammer, Dietrich.
 [Sprachlose Kind. English]
 Speaking honestly with sick and dying children and
adolescents : unlocking the silence / Dietrich Niethammer ;
foreword by Christoph Schmeling-Kludas, foreword by
Ruprecht Nitschke ; translated by Victoria W. Hill.
   p. ; cm.
 Includes bibliographical references and index.
 ISBN-13: 978-1-4214-0455-4 (hdbk. : alk. paper)
 ISBN-10: 1-4214-0455-9 (hdbk. : alk. paper)
 ISBN-13: 978-1-4214-0456-1 (pbk. : alk. paper)
 ISBN-10: 1-4214-0456-7 (pbk. : alk. paper)
 I. Title.
 [DNLM: 1. Child. 2. Terminally Ill—psychology.
3. Adolescent. 4. Attitude to Death. 5. Physician-Patient
Relations. WS 200]
 LC classification not assigned
 618.92'0029—dc23   2011029812

A catalog record for this book is available from the British
Library.

*Special discounts are available for bulk purchases of this book. For
more information, please contact Special Sales at 410-516-6936 or
specialsales@press.jhu.edu.*

Contents

Foreword

Christoph Schmeling-Kludas, M.D.
Professor of Medicine, Psychosomatic Clinic, Ginsterhof

How do healthy and terminally ill children and adolescents deal with the topic of death and dying? That is the question at the heart of this book. The starting point is an analysis of the available literature, beginning with Freud's work. The book owes its development to the special background of its author: Dietrich Niethammer is a prominent representative of pediatric oncology in an era characterized by unparalleled advancements, successes to which he substantially contributed. Yet he remained sensitive to the emotional situation of his patients, often very young and terminally ill, at a time when the "soullessness of high-tech medicine" was widely and justly deplored.

Children arouse not only in their parents but also in their caregivers the need to protect and save them. It is difficult for them to endure situations in which it is unclear whether their efforts will succeed. Staying by the side of children and adolescents who are sick, not withdrawing from them, and carrying out the necessary diagnostic and therapeutic measures with empathy and affection is already a great deal. From the individual case studies in the book, it is clear that Niethammer went much further: he allowed himself to encounter the children on a personal level. He permitted his young patients to touch him emotionally, to question his ideas, to criticize him, and to show him new ways of doing things. This was only possible by achieving a special kind of psychological integration. As a doctor, Niethammer had at his disposal a scientific point of view with the requisite detachment. But at the same time he showed real empathy for the children and adolescents for whom he and other pediatric oncologists were developing therapeutic approaches that were becoming more invasive and sometimes life-threatening and that demanded everything a human being could tolerate and cope with. Perhaps because the new therapeutic strategies were so successful, Niethammer, himself the father of three sons, was able to endure this situation throughout his professional life. He put into practice the concept of psychosomatic medicine developed by Thure von Uexküll, the doyen of German and European psychosomatic medicine who died in 2004. He was able to do this even in a medical specialty that from a psychotherapeutic perspective involves particularly difficult emotional work. If everyone practiced medicine as Niethammer does, psychosomatic medicine as a separate specialty could be done away with, just as Uexküll had always wished.

The process set in motion by his concept of medical practice allowed Niethammer to overcome the position, believed universally well into the 1970s, that we should never talk with children about their illness and approaching death. He came to the conclusion, at first haltingly and then more and more forthrightly, that open communication, radical honesty, and the promise never to lie to the patient made it easier for adolescents and even very young children to cope with the threat of death and the necessary therapies. This is also true for those who must recognize at some point that they are dying.

Since this involvement, which has lasted his entire professional life, Niethammer is now investigating what the pertinent scientific disciplines have found out about the ideas of children and adolescents relating to death and dying and what conclusions were drawn based on these studies. Beginning with the classic writings of psychoanalysis, he examines and evaluates the literature of developmental psychology as well as pediatrics, sometimes with surprising results. Primarily on the basis of clinical experience, other authors concluded, as he had, that an understanding of death and dying appears much earlier in human development than had long been postulated. It has also become clear that we must recognize the large individual differences among children of the same age and differentiate between ideas about death in healthy and sick children. Previously held views based in developmental psychology about the age at which humans are able to imagine death and dying and how they do so must obviously be revised.

As a practitioner of psychosomatics and psychotherapy, I am hopeful that this book will find many readers in oncology and clinical medicine as well as in developmental psychology. Because of the vividness with which existential human questions are treated, reading the book provides personal enrichment in any case—as long as the reader is prepared to confront the reality that burdens us on every page: the death of children and adolescents.

Foreword

Ruprecht Nitschke, M.D.
Professor Emeritus of Pediatrics, University of Oklahoma
Health Sciences Center

Dietrich Niethammer, a widely recognized pediatric hematologist and on-cologist, professor emeritus at the University of Tübingen in Germany, states in the introduction to his book that the psychological guidance of a dying person is one of the physician's basic tasks. In his words: "This task is just as challenging as making a difficult diagnosis or implementing a complex ther-apy." His book addresses the question of psychological guidance for a child with a life-threatening disease. He had a haunting experience as an extern, in the mid-1960s, while caring for a twelve-year-old girl with advanced can-cer. She had become silent, refusing to communicate with anybody. This ex-perience led to the title of his book, *Das Sprachlose Kind* (The speechless child). Instead of this image of a lost child, the title of the English translation envisions the author's intent: *Speaking Honestly with Sick and Dying Children and Adolescents: Unlocking the Silence*. The frequently observed silence of these children is a product of fear of the unknown and lack of information about the disease afflicting them. The caregivers were unable to talk about the chil-dren's concerns. This situation could have been prevented by communicating openly with these children. Since the 1970s the author and his team have been telling them the truth about their disease, diagnosis, and prognosis and giving them the chance to express their thoughts, fears, and concerns. As a result, these young patients do not die in isolation. Niethammer's objectives for this book are, first, to familiarize the reader with the open approach and, second, to investigate why psychological guidance of a dying child was so long neglected in the last century and is still not fully accepted.

Niethammer reviews English, French, and German publications about children with terminal diseases. The first chapters of his book are concerned with how a child deals with illness, followed by a chapter about the physi-cian's traditionally paternalistic attitude and the importance of patient au-tonomy. The last four chapters consist of a historical review of various concepts of death in healthy and chronically sick children and a discussion of truth-telling and decisionmaking as it relates to children with advanced terminal diseases.

The author presents his data by outlining information gathered from the literature as well as from his personal observations. He reports on his own successful interventions and misjudgments.

In analyzing the publications, Niethammer presents convincing data for using the open communication style with children. M. Bluebond-Langner and A. DeCicco, cited by him, came to the same conclusion in their chapter "Children's Views of Death," an excellent and detailed analysis of this topic that appeared in *Oxford Textbook of Palliative Care of Children* (2006).

Many of Niethammer's comments and observations mirror my own experiences in caring for children with cancer over a forty-year career. One incident concerned a four-and-a-half-year-old boy whose advanced disease resisted further treatment. I suggested we tell him the facts, including his inevitable death. The parents refused, so I encouraged them to talk about it at home with him. They left the conference wondering how a doctor could encourage them to talk to a four-year-old about death.

Several weeks later, the boy came into the kitchen asking his mother, "Why can't I run like everybody else?" She then told him that his leukemia therapy had ceased to work and that he would die. She continued: "Do you know what will happen when you die?"

"What?" he asked.

"You will go to heaven."

"What is heaven?"

"The place where God lives."

"Who is God?" The conversation went on a little longer, and later, at bedtime, his stepfather asked him, "Would you like to go fishing with God?"

"Yes, Daddy, but does God have fishing poles?"

"I don't know, but if he doesn't, he can catch them with his hands."

"Won't the snapping turtles bite him?"

"Andrew, there are no turtles that bite in heaven!" After discussing the chance to paint a rainbow with God, his stepfather asked him, "Is there anything else?"

"Yes. Mommy, will Snow White be there?"

"Yes, Andrew."

"That's all I wanted to know. Good night!"

The stepfather reported this story to me, amazed and deeply relieved. Again and again I was astonished at the capabilities of dying children. They not only understand their future but also make plans for the time remaining to them, for instance taking vacations, visiting friends, attending school, giving away their most cherished belongings, and expressing concern for the welfare of their loved ones after they die. These behaviors have enormous implications for those who are guiding and supporting the children. They also facilitate the grief process for both the children and their survivors.

American readers may occasionally be surprised by observations or statements that reveal cultural differences between Germany and America. An example of this is chapter 7, "The 'Precociously Mature' Child." The concept of premature spiritual/emotional development is rarely discussed by American investigators. These differences do not detract from the value of this book, however. Its content is pertinent for cancer patients as well as those with other chronic illnesses that become terminal. I sincerely hope that this book will find an attentive audience among caregivers for sick and dying children: medical professionals, psychologists, social workers, and other professionals as well as laypersons.

Niethammer challenges the medical profession to become more familiar with the thoughts and behaviors of chronically ill children and to develop psychological guidelines of care. For example, criteria need to be developed for the identification of children with progressive disease who may not tolerate or understand the hard news that they will die soon. Also, guidelines are necessary for the crucial point at which a child's prognosis changes. These guidelines would include a meeting to clarify the new expectations and options. It would address the changes in treatment plans and open a dialogue about the child's wishes for this final stage. Finally, a sophisticated evaluation of all children and families who participate in this dialogue would enhance our understanding and lead to improved interventions. It is obvious that well-designed prospective programs are needed.

This book serves another useful purpose in bringing attention to the problems surrounding the physicians' role and obligations in today's world, considering the financial realities. Psychological support programs require a physician's commitment and time, which are often inadequately reimbursed. Another impediment to the development of Niethammer's type of program is purely practical. Treating childhood cancer from a medical standpoint is complex. It leaves little time or opportunity for physicians, who frequently have not been trained in psychological guidance, to develop supportive programs. Therefore, close collaboration among medical team members, psychologists, and social workers increases the potential for optimal and holistic treatment programs for children with cancer.

Preface

During the first half of the 1960s I was completing a residency in a children's hospital. There I met a dying child, a nine-year-old girl suffering from cancer who no longer spoke with anyone and finally, one night, died completely alone. Today, forty years later, I still remember well the unpleasant feeling that crept over me afterward. Something about the situation wasn't right, but I didn't know yet what it was. This child, who stared wide-eyed at anyone who came into her room and remained stubbornly silent, was almost unbearable. She didn't even respond to questions.

During my years in medical school, death and dying were never mentioned in any of the lectures. At the most, someone occasionally pointed out that under no circumstances should we enlighten patients about their bad situation. As we accompanied our teachers on their hospital rounds, we often experienced how they wove numerous Latin expressions into their explanations in order to remain incomprehensible to laypersons (the patients). Often they closed their monologue with the remark, "extra muros," which was intended to make it clear to us that anything further was to be discussed outside the hospital room. When I began my training in pediatrics at a German university hospital in the early 1970s after a three-year research fellowship in the United States, this situation had not changed at all. Among other things, I was soon assigned the care of children with cancer and given the following guidelines to take along with me: (1) children are not to be informed about what kind of illness they have, and the diagnosis is never to be stated; (2) children's questions should only be answered if they have nothing to do with the diagnosis or its potential consequences; and (3) the topics of death and dying should be avoided under all circumstances.

The result was that we consistently lied to the children. Fortunately— fortunately for us, that is—they soon stopped asking questions. We failed to understand that the children had perceived how pointless it was for them to ask questions, so they soon stopped. And so we continued our charade. At the time I repeatedly encountered children who no longer spoke with anyone and who died a lonely death. It was a time in which over 80 percent of children and adolescents with cancer died of their malignant disease. But the first successful treatments were emerging, so the majority of patients was transferred to hospitals in which doctors specialized in the new forms of therapy. The result was that the number of young people with cancer in our care grew steadily. And the number of "silent" children increased as well.

As two or three years passed, this began to seem more and more bizarre to me, until one day a twelve-year-old girl with leukemia opened my eyes. She told me clearly and distinctly that she knew what she had and that she would die of it. An intensive dialogue between her and her deeply shocked young doctor ensued, during which I tried to make it clear that her assumption wasn't necessarily correct, since effective therapies had developed in the meantime. Several intensive conversations followed, and I was surprised at how openly she talked about her situation and her problems with me. This occurrence, it seemed to me, pointed to the right approach, and I began to talk openly with the other children too. I experienced how the sick children and adolescents began to open up. I learned from them that they did not want to be lied to and that they almost always saw through our charade. And soon there were no more silent children. When I took over the Hematology-Oncology Division of the Department of Pediatrics at the University Hospital in Tübingen, I implemented the principle of honesty with my new team. I can still remember how much resistance I encountered, especially from the experienced members of the team. But after six months the situation had eased, since most of the team members had experienced for themselves what a relief it was to be able to give up the charade.

In short, from then on the children in Tübingen were no longer silent. In the years that followed, I frequently came across publications that appeared to confirm my position with regard to openness. And fortunately I met colleagues like my friend Ed Forman, pediatric oncologist at Brown University in Providence, Rhode Island, who thought exactly as I did. But my responsibilities as director of a hospital left me too little time for reading, so for a long time the pioneering publication by Joel Vernick and Myron Karon and the articles by Ruprecht Nitschke's group in Oklahoma City escaped my notice. They provided evidence that my ideas were correct, since their authors had recognized before I did that we should not lie to children. Nitschke was actually the son of one of my predecessors in Tübingen; I had known him as a young student, and he made a strong impression on me at the time. Not until the 1990s did a productive dialogue develop between us; it is described in this book in some detail.

During the last twenty years I have asked myself again and again why it took so long for us to recognize that we need to talk openly with sick children. How did it happen that this insight became the foundation of caregiving so slowly, as late as the end of the twentieth century? During the first seven or eight decades of the century, medicine clung stubbornly to the opinion that children don't think about death and dying, the opinion that Sigmund Freud was the first to express. I resolved to look for the answers to these questions once my active professional life was over. As luck would have it, I was able to spend ten months at the Institute for Advanced Study in Berlin immediately after my retirement. With its library and its staff, it offered me a setting that was ideal for my purpose. Not many doctors before me had the good fortune to spend a year at the institute with more than forty scholars from all over the world and from many different disciplines—primarily in the humanities. In this stimulating atmosphere, I went searching for clues, and the results are here in this book. I found answers to my questions. I hope I have succeeded in presenting the results of my research in such a way that the reader understands the message: Children think about death and dying, and they want to talk about it, above all when they themselves are affected.

Acknowledgments

I would like to express my heartfelt thanks to the financial sponsors of the Institute for Advanced Study in Berlin (both federal and state governments) and to the selection committee that invited me to Berlin. I would also like to thank the staff at the institute, who made my stay an uninterrupted pleasure. I am also grateful to my co-fellows, who contributed to a stimulating atmosphere and were always ready for discussion and conversation. As representatives of the group as a whole, I mention a few names with whom my exchange of ideas was especially intensive and who were very helpful to me in my project: Robert Aronowitz, specialist in internal medicine in Philadelphia; Ingolf Dalferth, Protestant theologian from Zurich; Judit Frigyesi and her son Ben, musicologists from Israel; Carla Hesse and her husband Thomas Laqueur, historians from Berkeley; Mordechai Kremnitzer, attorney, and his wife Rivka Feldhay, historian of science, from Israel. The institute provided me the wonderful opportunity of inviting my friend Ed Forman, pediatric oncologist at Brown University, to participate as a guest. Over a period of many years we have shared ideas about interacting with seriously ill children and adolescents, and I am extremely grateful to him for the in-depth discussions about my project during his stay in Berlin.

I would also like to thank my colleagues in Tübingen who made it possible for me to put the concepts of caregiving I had developed through the years into practice and prove them correct. Our ongoing exchange of ideas and our close collaboration for the benefit of severely ill children and adolescents were always a source of great satisfaction for me. Over the years, my colleagues were almost always willing to follow me on the path to further improvements in the holistic care of severely ill children and adolescents and their families. There are too many to name, but I would like to thank in particular psychologist and psychoanalyst Manon Hoffmeister, a colleague in my department during my first years in Tübingen. The theoretical concepts behind what had previously been my intuitive and practical approach to caring for and supporting the children and their families became clear to me in the course of many conversations with her.

I am grateful to Wulf Bertram of Schattauer Verlag for his willingness to publish this book and to his colleague Marie Teltscher for her very competent and helpful editorial work. I also thank Bernd Hontschik for his valuable advice. I very much appreciate the financial support from the Jung-Stiftung für Wissenschaft und Forschung in Hamburg, without which the book would not have been published.

I am grateful to Jacqueline Wehmueller of the Johns Hopkins University Press, who made the publication of this book in the United States possible and helped to shape it, and to Victoria W. Hill for her careful and skilled translation.

I owe a debt of gratitude to Dietlinde Niethammer, my wife of more than forty years. She listened patiently to me throughout my professional life and also asked many critical questions; she always gave me strength when I came close to despair over the fates of the young people who were dying. She also provided critical support in the preparation of this manuscript. Medical students often asked me how it was possible to survive work as difficult as that of a pediatric oncologist. I always answer that first of all, you can learn a great deal, and second, you need a dependable partner with whom you can talk about everything. Besides, I am convinced that we gain much more from the children than we can ever invest in them.

I have learned an immense amount from the seriously ill children and their families who were in my care during more than three decades. I am grateful to fate for placing me in my life's work, which also happened to be connected to major therapeutic advances in the treatment of cancer. So I dedicate this book to the children and adolescents who were and are suffering from serious illness. I hope this book can help others assist young people who are sick and in need.

Speaking Honestly with Sick
and Dying Children and Adolescents

CHAPTER ONE

Introduction

Death must have occupied people's thoughts from the very beginning. At some stage in the development from animal to human, we became conscious of death. Since then, in our religious and mystical thought and, to a lesser extent, in our everyday lives, we have been dealing with our fears and reflections on life after death. Death has always been an important subject in both philosophy and psychoanalysis.

The Greek philosopher Plato portrayed the philosopher Socrates as thinking extensively about death (Guardini 1956). But representatives of various fields of study differ greatly in the metaphysical and biological concepts they use. For the psychoanalyst Sigmund Freud, for example, death is the final goal toward which life moves. But for the philosopher Martin Heidegger it represents a continuous threat. Of course, none of these concepts is based on empirical data (Bromberg et al. 1933).

For a long time, medicine did not seriously confront the question of the role that death plays for children. There are probably several reasons for this avoidance. First, for many centuries, even millennia, the death of children was an everyday event. The healing arts and, later, medical science often had nothing available to counter it. The death of children was more or less accepted as an inevitable occurrence. Not until the end of the nineteenth century did doctors begin to comprehend that there might be ways to decrease the incidence of child mortality. Their approach to dealing with the problem, however, was limited to the realm of medicine and social medicine and primarily addressed newborns and young children. Beginning in the second half of the twentieth century, seriously ill children survived later and later into life until eventually they died of their illness. At this point some doctors began to ask themselves exactly what meaning death had for children.

By the first decades of the twentieth century, psychoanalysts and developmental psychologists had begun to study concepts of death in healthy children. But it took them a long time to acknowledge that children were able to think critically about death. Only in the 1960s did clinical practitioners begin to grapple with the death of children and with children's own understanding of the process. Until then, psychoanalysts and developmental psychologists had primarily studied healthy children; at most, sick children would get only a passing mention in the discussion. Occasionally, they expressed the thought that having a severe illness might influence children's thoughts on the subject. But during the first half of the twentieth century, psychoanalysts and developmental psychologists attached little importance to this question. No one considered it necessary to look for an answer. Only after much time had passed were any conclusions drawn from these reflections.

This book describes the progression from Freud's first statements about children's concepts of death (1900, 1913, 1915) to the conclusions gradually drawn from thinking critically about sick children, conclusions that should increasingly determine our current approach. Above all, I think it is important to develop a fundamental concept of how children think about death and dying, relying on the often contradictory studies by a wide range of authors. With this literature as a foundation, I intend to elaborate guidelines for doctors' daily practice, supported by my own lengthy experience with seriously ill and dying children. Detailed guidelines, however, falling outside the framework of this book, will be published separately.

A potential criticism might be that in contrast to the objectives of psychoanalysts or developmental psychologists, my objectives slight theoretical concepts about children in favor of the children's own thinking and knowledge. That may be the case, but in my clinical practice I have always been interested in understanding what sick children find important about death and dying. Schematic concepts such as those posited by Jean Piaget, for example, are of limited utility. They should play a role in interactions with sick people only insofar as they clarify factors that may otherwise be confusing for the physicians involved.

In 1995 the general studies program in Tübingen hosted a conference entitled "Dying with Dignity" (Jens and Küng 1995). The German studies specialist and rhetorician Walter Jens and the Catholic theologian Hans Küng intended to use this event to clarify their position on active help in dying, as has been legal in the Netherlands for some time. They called for the introduction of the same kind of active procedure in Germany as well, since in their opinion a self-determined death would help ensure a dignified and humane death. In my counterproposal at the closing session, I related the story of a young girl, Jutta, ill with cancer, whom I had encountered as a medical student in the mid-1960s when I was doing a rotation in a pediatric clinic. On that occasion, I was confronted with a dying child for the first time.

I recounted this story then to make the point that this kind of death was undignified and inhumane and that an injection would not have changed anything. I expressed the opinion that a person's death is always undignified and inhumane if they are left alone during the transition to death.

JUTTA WAS A twelve-year-old girl whose body was riddled with tumors. She was already so weak that she could no longer get out of bed. Her body was reduced to a skeleton, and she refused all nourishment. Only her large, dark eyes still seemed alive; she would direct them at a new arrival, only to look quickly past him or her into empty space if the visitor were to speak to her. Jutta no longer spoke with anyone, not with the doctors, not with the nurses, and not with her parents, during their twice-weekly visiting hours in which they tried desperately to radiate good cheer. All of us found Room No. 3 unbearable. We only went in when our duties demanded it, and we would always leave as quickly as possible. We found that our words were catching in our throats more and more often. One morning Jutta was dead; no one was with her when she died. During her rounds, the night nurse had discovered the girl dead in her bed. I was relieved at her death, and at the same time I was ashamed. Jutta had already been removed from the ward under cover of night. We never talked about her again; it was as if she had never existed.

Even as a student I was certain that I had witnessed a horrible death in this case, that something had gone wrong. We had learned nothing about how to deal with death and the dying in medical school, and the textbooks were also silent on the subject. I also can't recall that any of our teachers ever broached the topic. As a result, what had happened to the little girl remained unclear to me for a long time. Later, as a young doctor, I was to see many people, both adults and children, die without a word—alone, abandoned, often in a tiled bathroom or a storage room, since there were hardly any single rooms in hospitals at the time. Over and over again, I saw Jutta before me, sitting on the edge of a bathtub or on an upside-down bucket, with her great big eyes. There had been only one occasion when I tried desperately to talk with her that she didn't immediately look away.

After I became involved in the care and treatment of children with cancer in the beginning of the 1970s, I encountered such silent children over and over again. In 1978 the psychologist Georg Wolff asked why children with cancer are silent. But it would be a long time until behavior toward sick children and adolescents in routine medical practice changed and the terrible silence in the hospitals became the exception rather than the norm.

By the mid-1970s it became clear to me and certain other pediatricians that lack of information was probably the main reason for the behavior of these dying children. The children were not allowed to learn anything about the nature of their illness and the threats it presented, and talking with them about their probable death was absolutely forbidden. According to the general orthodoxy, the only questions that should be answered were those that had nothing to do with these topics. And because we evaded the children's questions about illness and death, the children soon stopped asking, since they could see through our behavior. They gave up their attempts to converse with us. Based on my experiences with sick children, I slowly began to change my behavior; over time, my answers to their questions became increasingly candid. Today, I am certain that, as doctors, we should not lie to sick children and adolescents if we want to provide them the necessary support during the transition to death. Along with many others, I finally understood: it is wrong to assume that children do not contemplate their illness or death itself.

The root of this false supposition was probably the helplessness pediatricians have long felt in being unable to provide effective therapy. So this assumed lack of interest in children was comforting, since you were not obliged to talk about these facts with the children and adolescents. The general attempt in modern life to make death invisible certainly also played an important role, since for a long time we didn't talk with dying adults about their situation either. That this was probably handled differently in past centuries is covered later in the book. The dictum attributed to Christoph Wilhelm Hufeland, a renowned physician of the early nineteenth century, "He who names death, brings death," had been accepted as the doctor's highest precept for far too long. So too the assertion, repeated like a mantra, that "We must never take away the patient's hope." These two assertions have one thing in common: you don't talk with the sick person about his or her impending death. For a long time, these convictions kept doctors from a proper discussion about death and dying. The books of Swiss psychiatrist Elisabeth Kübler-Ross (1969, 1985) first called the public's attention to the phenomenon of dying, with the result that doctors could no longer avoid the issue.

Although the insight that we have to deal more openly with children and adolescents has continued to gain acceptance, it remains unclear to many doctors just how far they should go. As recently as 2004, the respected *New England Journal of Medicine* published an article by a Swedish working group (Kreicbergs et al. 2004) in which the authors reported on interviews with 449 parents who had lost a child to cancer. Only a third had talked to their children about death at any time, not necessarily in close chronological proximity to the death; almost none of the parents regretted this. Two-thirds never spoke with their children about this subject, and just under one-third of them had regrets about it. The authors concluded that parents should be encouraged to have such conversations; I believe that current research suggests even more strongly that they should have done so. The published reactions to this article were similarly noncommittal or even rather negative.

The pediatrician Lawrence Wolfe pointed out in an editorial that many children probably know more than is generally assumed and that this population-based study conveys a clear message about the emotional experience of parents with a dying child (Wolfe 2004). The children's needs did not play a substantial role in either the study or the comments. One reader's letter pointed out that open communication is often helpful but that there are also many counterexamples (Davies 2005). And the author of another letter was quite clearly against spelling things out, because "it is egoistical to avoid our own feelings of regret by exposing a child to the potential fears, sadness, or alienation connected to the reality of dying" (Tanvetyanon 2005). So it is not surprising that there are many doctors today who express the opinion that we should make patients aware of the seriousness of their illness and then qualify their opinion with a "but" and cite counterarguments that speak against honesty in this or that particular case. This is an escape hatch they can apparently use at any time with a clear conscience. And so many patients become just such a special case, and many doctors do not even realize that they are actually viewing all of their patients as "special cases." Many reports from family members of deceased patients attest to this fact.

As a university professor, I knew many students who were unable to imagine how anyone could become a pediatric oncologist. It became clear in the course of many conversations how afraid the young people were that they would not be up to the challenges of caring for seriously ill or even dying children. Paracelsus himself was already aware, I always replied, that understanding the "how" is the crucial foundation that enables doctors to do the right thing for patients and to provide them adequate support. In order to treat an illness correctly, you have to understand its nature and its cause; in the same way, you have to be aware of a person's suffering and its causes in order to provide help. In fact, doctors can and must learn a great deal about what goes on in the affected children and their families, what problems the serious illness may trigger in them, and what is on their minds when they face death. This is something the seriously ill children and adolescents I treated and cared for over the years taught me.

In addition, we have to learn how to maintain the necessary distance from patients; after all, it is not our own children who are dying. Doctors who sympathize so much that they lose all distance to their patients are just as unhelpful as those who try to avoid being moved by what is happening so they can stand aloof from it. This is easier said than done, as every doctor probably has to learn the hard way. I remember well the many times I felt like running away; in other cases, I didn't want to accept that we had reached the end of therapeutic options. At some point I understood that it will never be possible to cure all sick children and adolescents and that, as a doctor, one must accept this fact. We must learn to understand that not abandoning a dying person is one of the fundamental duties of a doctor and that providing care does not stop with the end of therapy. This task is just as challenging as making a difficult diagnosis or implementing a complex therapy.

Not all doctors can master the problem of maintaining an appropriate distance in the same way. But they should have the courage to accept this reality and work in a different medical specialty as a consequence. This means not that they are bad doctors but that their talent most likely lies in a different area. Those with experience have to point the way for the inexperienced and keep an eye on them so that help is available if a breakdown threatens. A good team in which team members are concerned about each other and feel mutually responsible is helpful in this regard, as is supervision in the workplace and, last but not least, a good and stable life partner who can provide a firm foundation in difficult times.

Since we began speaking openly with children, we have learned a lot from them. Today they are no longer silent; instead they talk about their fears and worries. Knowing the fundamental nature of their illness and the danger it poses allows them to ask questions about things that concern them and to talk about everything that preoccupies them. With this book, I hope to address everyone involved with or interested in the care of seriously ill children and clarify why it has taken so long to convince the majority of doctors that interacting openly with them is the right approach. My motivation for investigating the issue was to discover the reasons for this delay, since on the one hand false ideas about children's level of knowledge have long been harmful to ill children and adolescents—and still are today. On the other hand, I hope to make the relationships clearer for the reader by describing this evolution. The goal is to encourage everyone involved in the care and support of seriously ill children and adolescents to confront the concept of openness and honesty, including its challenges, and act accordingly. How we should interact with seriously ill and dying children—guidelines that have grown out of encounters with patients—is beyond the scope of this book and must be covered elsewhere.

The ideas our predecessors and teachers had about how children think are interesting to us now, as are the conclusions they drew from them. At the same time, it is instructive to see how the representatives of various disciplines approached this set of problems. Developmental psychologists in particular have been interested in these questions for a long time, educators less so. It is also clear that medicine, particularly pediatric medicine, was especially slow to begin examining interactions with seriously ill and dying children. This discussion is far from over, as the example just cited from the *New England Journal of Medicine* makes all too clear. I also intend to discuss what concepts of death children and adolescents are able to develop at different ages and what consequences these differences have for their care. I hope a picture of the current state of knowledge about the problems addressed here will emerge.

It would be equally interesting to investigate why it took so long for us to begin informing dying adults about their situation; even today we do so only partially. But this book is about children and adolescents, and I am a pediatrician. Nevertheless, I won't hide my firm conviction that there are no major differences between children and adults with regard to the topics treated in this book. The questions on the minds of dying children don't differ fundamentally from the questions that concern adults. But I have met many internists who, like researchers in the field of pediatrics before them, view these issues very differently.

I want to emphasize one point at the outset, because it has influenced my approach and my attitude toward the authors I cite. I am deeply convinced of the importance of truth. We as doctors cannot lie to sick children and adolescents, not even when we have bad news for them or when death is imminent. They must be able to rely on this honesty. It will also give truth value to our positive statements, something patients in these difficult situations desperately need. Evasive answers are lies too! Although I am not the only one to take this position, it is clear to me that I find myself at the extreme end of a spectrum of attitudes where not informing the patient is at the opposite end. With respect to this issue, I have been heavily influenced by my many experiences with children.

We must never forget that dying is a stage of life—albeit the final one. So care for the dying also means care for the living. Not until the child entrusted to us

I WILL NEVER forget the dialogue in which a twelve-year-old boy asked me for the first time if dying hurts. I hesitated with my answer, because I was taken completely by surprise when this question was fired off in the middle of a conversation about a game we had just finished, and I had no clever answer on the tip of my tongue. The boy noticed my hesitation and said, "Professor, you promised you would never lie!" Stalling for time, I said, "You know, I haven't died yet." "I know that," was the child's somewhat impatient answer. "But what do you think?" "You know," I answered, "I have sat by the bedside of dying children many times, and I never got the impression that dying itself was painful." "That's good," was his concluding comment. My answer had reassured him. This question, of concern to everyone who knows they will have to die, is raised again and again, and I would repeat this answer often.

has died does the care cease and the doctor must leave the child. But the parents and siblings live on, and they need care after the death of their child, their sister, or their brother. Of course, we have to ask whether there is a "right way" to die (Silvermann 2000). Freud (1915) already pointed out that no one can think constantly about his or her own death, an issue A. Weisman revisited in 1972. Even people suffering from a fatal illness cannot constantly live with the thought that in the end they will die of it. That would make life in the present unbearable. According to Weisman, we live with a "middle knowledge"—that is, we are aware of our own death, but it remains in the background. That is not the same as denial; it means instead that we have to live with contradictory philosophies and the flexibility to move freely among them. According to Silvermann (2000), "Whether we have understood something adequately must be tested in the world as it is and not as we would like it to be."

Weisman does not believe that death always follows an orderly course. Instead, we have to help the dying find a death that is suitable for them. Children in particular must have the opportunity to create a reality that they can sustain until the end. And we must help them in this process. The ideas that children develop with their imaginations have an important role to play here. That doesn't mean, however, that reality is nonexistent.

Discussions of active help in dying as it is practiced in Holland and Switzerland are also occurring in Germany (Jens and Küng 1995). Inherent in this practice is the risk of making only the final act of dying the focal point. In 1978 Lofland described this trend as "the death movement," and others raised the alarm about it as well (Lofland 1978). She pointed out that modern medicine, with its advanced techniques, is in a position to define people as "dying people" long before death actually occurs. These people no longer have a social function and thus have to live for lengthy periods virtually as unpersons. Lofland makes clear that people caring for someone who is dying should focus on life, that they must concentrate not on the quality of death but on the quality of life until the actual occurrence of death.

And so this book about death is actually a book about the life of children and adolescents at the end of their human existence—a life full of despair and suffering but often full of cheerfulness, love, and devotion. A century after Freud's first statements at the beginning of the twentieth century (1913), we have come a long way in our understanding of how young people who are seriously ill think, and we can assist them much better in their suffering. It seems we have come full circle to the point that Swiss poet Gottfried Keller had already reached in 1878. In *The Governor of Greifensee,* one of his Zurich novellas, he describes the comforting behavior of the governor toward a dying child, in this context probably with the intention of characterizing the worthy man:

> Once, a neighbor's little ten-year-old son lay dying of an incurable illness, and neither the encouragement of the pastor nor that of his parents was able to console the child in his pain and his fear of death, for he would have liked so much to live. So the governor sat down next to his bed, calmly smoking his pipe, and talked to him in such simple and fitting words of the hopelessness of his situation, of the necessity of pulling himself together and suffering for a short time, but also of the blissful, unchanging calm that would be granted him as a patient and pious little boy, of the love and sympathy that he, a stranger, felt for him, so that from that hour on the child changed, bearing his sufferings with cheerful patience until he was in fact released by death.

This depiction may seem a bit too idyllic to some readers, but Gottfried Keller does make it clear in this passage what the dying child needed.

CHAPTER TWO

Children, Sickness, and Death

For many decades psychoanalysts and developmental psychologists tried to identify concepts of death and dying in healthy children only. I believe this approach is fundamentally wrong if the goal is to learn something about what seriously ill or dying children think. So in this chapter I would like to sketch briefly, for the benefit of the uninformed reader, what serious illness means for a child. I hope that this knowledge will make my critique of many researchers' procedures and results more understandable.

If we are interested in finding out how children deal with death and dying, we first have to ask under what circumstances children die. Once we try to answer that question, we see that the answer may be more complex for children and adolescents than for adults, since different age groups have different characteristics. We must also understand what becoming seriously ill means for a child or adolescent. Surely the special thing about childhood is that there are no long-term plans for the future, especially for young children. In consequence, dying does not create the feeling that things already planned must be left unfinished, as it does for adults. But the feeling of having to deal with something before dying definitely does arise, even in young children.

Illnesses differ greatly in how they influence children's lives. To understand these influences better, we need to call to mind the various types of illness. Acute illnesses may be harmless and transitory, they may be accompanied by substantial impairment, or they may be life-threatening. There are also chronic illnesses—congenital or acquired disorders—that may or may not progress and damage children's quality of life in the long run. Some chronic illnesses progress in phases with intervals in which the child is impaired only slightly, if at all. Among the chronic illnesses we must include those that are incurable and eventually lead to death. Enumerating the types of illness clarifies how differently children may be affected by them.

Communication with children of any age is impossible or extremely limited if they die in an intensive care unit, usually unconscious, after an accident or a brief, extremely serious illness. In this circumstance the medical team's assistance has to be limited to medical problems, and it is the immediate family of the children who need emotional support. Often the grandparents are as deeply affected as the children's parents, and they should not be forgotten. In modern medicine, the question of whether the dying child may qualify as an organ donor can arise. For many parents, this situation encompasses a new and additional dimension that is difficult to deal with. The team needs to be especially sensitive in such circumstances. Parents may categorically reject this idea, or they may feel a certain sense of relief that the child's death might become meaningful in that the organ donation allows another sick child to live.

The situation is not much different in neonatal medicine, when especially tiny premature babies, as well as newborns and infants who have been badly damaged for various reasons, die. Here again, it is the family members who desperately need support. Here too, someone dies in intensive care. Often the process of dying is overshadowed by existential questions, particularly when it comes to the decision to discontinue efforts to save a badly damaged child. In this case the decision to discontinue treatment, rather than a possible organ donation, may cause a major moral dilemma for the parents.

Young infants, who most often die as a result of an acute illness, are not in a position to express their wishes and ideas in a concrete way. This situation changes with increasing age, as children's capabilities for communicating and expressing themselves sharpen, and at the same time illnesses that lead to death tend to run a lengthier course. So older children, like adults, have the possibility of coming to grips with their illness and eventually with death as well. Due to a lack of therapeutic options in the past, serious illnesses ran a brief course and led quickly to death. For example, during the first two-thirds of the last century, children with cancer often died just a few days or weeks after diagnosis. Children with pneumonia or other infections often succumbed quickly to their disease. Today almost 70 percent of children and adolescents with cancer survive, and those who can't be cured often die after a long course of illness, sometimes lasting several years. And death from pneumonia or meningitis has fortunately become a rarity in our society. To give another example, patients born with cystic fibrosis now usually live into their thirties or forties; in the 1970s very few of them survived until their tenth birthday. Other congenital illnesses as well, such as those affecting the nervous or muscular system, end in death only after a number of years.

And all children and adolescents, if they die after living with their illness for a long time, have acquired a lot of experience. They have to deal with their parents' worries day in and day out, as well as with the problems, side effects, and consequences of their illness and the therapeutic measures used. They have a lot of time to think about everything and gather information— something that has become easy in the age of the internet, at least for older children and adolescents. And they have gotten to know other children with the same illness who have died in the meantime. During the lonely nights in the hospital, where many of them stay again and again until it becomes a kind of second home, they talk over their problems with their fellow sufferers. And they have to cope with the limitations the illness imposes on their daily lives—on play, on school, on their education, or, later, on finding a life partner. Although the treatment of a child with diabetes may appear to be proceeding normally now that there are clear standards and excellent care in treatment centers, we should not overlook the fact that these children's lives are by no means "normal." "I always have to take my disease with me, to school, to parties, and on vacation," as a fifteen-year-old girl once described her situation. And in fact she does have to watch her diet, measure her blood sugar daily, and give herself insulin injections. She added pensively, "The children who have cancer can at least forget about it at times like that and leave it at home."

The journey of life does not always lead in a straight line toward death for children and adolescents with severe chronic illnesses; many of them live with their illness long enough to see adulthood. But at some point they must confront that moment in their life when the imminence of death can no longer be overlooked. And all of these children try to come to grips with their death. Well into the 1970s they could not do this openly because adults didn't permit it, in the belief that children do not think about death. Those children died very much alone, as children still do when there is no one who communicates adequately with them. The fate of chronically ill children should be of particular concern to us, as should the options we have for helping them cope with problems caused by their illness.

As a result of their illness, these children must allow others more or less to control their lives, a situation they may grow to perceive as disagreeable. For us humans, each step we take toward achieving independence in a wide range of activities is a milestone on the way to developing our identity. Some children struggle against outside control and may come to be called "difficult" patients. Others resign themselves to their fates without resistance. The regression forced on these children from outside may cause them to lose skills recently acquired or not yet firmly established, skills that may have to be relearned after the illness, especially in the case of toddlers. This forced regression is particularly serious during adolescence, when the process of separating from parents that has already begun is drastically interrupted by the illness.

Forced immobility due to prescribed bed rest is also a big problem for many children, generally affecting them much more than specific dietary requirements. It has been noted that sick children go to bed voluntarily if they feel bad. But children, especially young children, often don't feel impaired by a high fever. So bed rest prescribed for fever will undoubtedly lead to conflict between the reluctant child and his or her worried parents, who of course want to follow the doctor's orders in the best interests of their child.

Worried parents also have a tendency to impose restrictions that are not really necessary. Often enough doctors accommodate their desire to do something additional, since the essential things are usually done by the professional caregivers, the doctors and nurses. Parents feel good when they can actively participate in this kind of situation. But doctors and parents should always question the usefulness of additional restrictions.

The disruption of family structure brought about by their illness is often a big problem for sick children. The parents' behavior toward the sick child, as well as toward the child's healthy siblings, changes in a major way, especially when the illness is life-threatening.

The enforced separation from friends and schoolmates brought about by the illness is also a problem for many children, especially when the illness is prolonged. In Germany, when children are sick for longer than six weeks, they are entitled to instruction in the hospital or at home. The hospital school, where patients are taught during a hospital stay in Germany, can relieve the situation considerably, as can visits by friends. It is not possible to deal extensively here with all the facets of interacting with and caring for sick children. The key factor, which I address extensively in the book, is honesty. Sick children must be informed about what will be happening to them. Children won't easily forget the assurance before blood is drawn that the needle won't hurt—a statement that, however well-intentioned, is often not accurate. Multiplied many times over, an experience like that will seriously disturb the children's sense of trust, making interactions with them much more difficult and transforming the illness into a traumatic experience.

Illness as Punishment

Illness is often misunderstood as punishment by sick children and adolescents, a fundamental point that we should not overlook. Every child has committed some kind of supposed or even real infraction in the period before the outbreak of their illness. Telling small lies or making excuses, concealing a bad grade, not doing what they were told or doing something forbidden, disobedience, and many other similar events happen daily in children's lives. They may burden healthy children briefly, but seldom do they develop into a serious problem. Anna Freud (1971) called them various forms of "misbehavior" for which there is a well-deserved punishment. Earlier, masturbation belonged to these offenses. It was a common view, often reinforced by religious teachers, that masturbation was a misguided sexual activity that weakened the organism and thus compromised the child's normal development. Today we know that this idea is nonsense.

The situation is quite different for sick children. Here the "infractions" carry a heavy weight, since from the children's viewpoint such offenses are to be punished—adults have often told them so. And so illness is viewed as punishment by many children, especially since in most cases the doctor can't tell them the real cause. Even when it is known (pathogens for a specific infectious disease, for example), the doctor can't explain why a particular child has contracted meningitis or rheumatic fever.

It doesn't take much imagination to see that an illness weighs heavily on children if they take it to be a punishment. The illness becomes a heavy burden, quite independent of its own direct effects, which are often hard enough on the child. In any case, such an idea weakens their strength to struggle against the illness and overcome it in a positive way; they develop a masochistic and passive attitude toward it. Occasionally, although fortunately very seldom, parents reinforce this sense of guilt, in part because they are desperately looking to identify a cause for the inexplicable.

Children do not always address the question of their guilt voluntarily. They may be too shy, they may not have developed enough trust in their new caregivers, or they may be afraid to confess to their parents an infraction that they regard as a catalyst. They may also fear the confirmation that they are being punished for an offense, and some children unconsciously prefer to live with uncertainty. At this point the doctor may be able to intervene in a helpful way. If we assume that virtually every sick child has similar ideas, we as doctors can initiate a discussion of this topic. One possibility is to ask the child directly. But the child may deny it, for the reasons described above. So it is usually helpful to say that you as a doctor have known other children who have had such thoughts. You will often observe that sick children are relieved to open up when they hear that the issue of punishment is also a problem for others. In routine clinical settings it has also proven helpful to mention the many people who committed serious offenses without becoming ill for that reason, even though they would have deserved it much more. That frequently makes sense to children. Often they can then put the issue of punishment to rest, opening a path for a positive approach to coping with the illness.

This suggests that the underlying reason for this view of punishment is a search for someone to blame. But as long as a person is to blame for his or her own misfortune, it is not really possible to deal satisfactorily with the illness. Mothers are especially likely to worry about the question of who is to blame, and they may occasionally transfer this concern to their child. I address the problem of mothers who feel guilt in more detail elsewhere. Doctors should be aware that if they cannot explain the cause of a serious illness, patients will see themselves as guilty, since there appears to be no other alternative.

CHAPTER THREE

Children in the Hospital

This chapter will address the question of what it means to children when they have to be admitted to the hospital. It is important to understand their feelings, because the majority of children and adolescents who die do so in a hospital. They have to deal intensively with this institution that sometimes functions as their second home for long periods.

Children and adolescents are usually admitted to the hospital only when they are so ill that they cannot be treated as outpatients. This is true for severe acute illnesses that usually lead to a single hospital stay and for chronic illnesses that may involve repeated stays lasting months, years, or possibly for life. Anna Freud and her collaborator Thesi Bergmann (1972) as well as Erich Stern (1957) described the significance of a severe illness for children in their books. Stern also dealt with the death of children. Dieter Bürgin's valuable book (1978), which will be discussed more thoroughly later, should also be noted.

For a child, admittance to a hospital for the first time will almost always be permanently associated with a traumatic experience. This was especially true when admittance meant a complete separation of children from their families, particularly their mothers. Until well into the 1970s, it was the practice in most hospitals to tell children, particularly very young ones, that their mother needed to leave the room for a moment to get something, after which the mother would not return. The little ones in particular would cry desperately for a long time before resigning themselves to the fact that crying was having no effect. Sooner or later they stopped crying and adapted to the strange surroundings and also to the new people with whom they had to deal. At that time, the length of stay was substantially longer than today, and there were many unmarried nurses in the hospitals whose primary purpose in life was their work. They were usually very committed to caring for the children; they tried to replace the absent mothers, and they were frequently quite successful in this. The children stopped crying and often became relatively calm. Although this reaction by the children to separation from their mothers had always been observable, it was in the 1940s and 1950s that it was first extensively described in the psychoanalytic literature (Freud 1943; Spitz 1947; Robertson and Bowlby 1952; Robertson 1953; Bowlby 1958, 1960a, 1960b). The English-speaking authors use the term *grief* for this phenomenon. The term is sometimes used to mean both the subjective experience following a loss and the psychological process it sets in motion (Freud 1943; Spitz 1947; Robertson 1953). In other studies the expression encompasses only the subjective experience (Bowlby 1960), which in the case of toddlers is naturally easier to judge and understand than the actual process of working through it.

During the first half of the twentieth century, most children's hospitals had no visiting hours at all; the danger of infection was used to justify the policy. In the second half of the century, it was often customary to allow parents to be with their children once or twice a week for a few hours. Other hospitals were designed so that parents could use an outside balcony surrounding the building to reach a window where they could at least establish eye contact with their children. In some hospitals there were even telephones they could use to communicate with their children from the balcony.

Visiting hours had one thing in common in every case: the moment the children discovered their mothers again, they began to scream and cry. For many nurses and doctors this behavior confirmed that it was much better for them if no parental visits were allowed. They did not understand that the children were in despair because their mother had vanished more or less magically after admission; this was certainly true for the younger children. Now, just as suddenly, the mother had reappeared (sometimes the father too). With their renewed crying, the children made clear their despair as well as their fear that their mother might once again disappear. And in fact many mothers would leave again after a short time, often without really saying goodbye, in the belief that furtively sneaking away was better for the child. This served primarily to make it easier for the mother, who could hardly bear the pain of another parting. However, sometimes the mother rushed to her child, delighted to see him or her again, but the child's attitude was wary, not least because he or she felt betrayed by the mother's behavior at the time of admission and was now distrustful. The mother of course would be very disappointed by this defensive behavior and often let the child know it. So a hospital stay often meant a psychic trauma for child and mother alike.

Fortunately, this procedure is now a thing of the past. Earlier, however, we subjected many children to traumatic experiences they would never forget. Today in most hospitals parents can stay overnight with their children. There are many legitimate reasons why mothers and fathers may need to go home at night—to care for healthy siblings, for example. In such cases, it is important for parents to say goodbye properly. It may lead to dramatic scenes of separation, and children may try with every means at their disposal to prevent the departure of the mother or to postpone it indefinitely. For young children, scenes like this are also not unusual at home, when it is time to go to bed. In both circumstances we have to be consistent and not give up because of the children's resistance; they need to learn how to deal with these necessary separations. We understand only too well that this consistent approach is especially difficult for parents leaving their children in the hospital. But we should never encourage parents to wait until the children have fallen asleep to leave, as a way of sparing everyone the pain of separation. At some point during the night a child may wake up and discover that he or she has been left alone. They are forced to interpret this as a deception, unless the mother had said she would not leave until the child had fallen asleep. The point here, as in many aspects of our interactions with children, is honesty. It is unacceptable to trick children or, even worse, to lie to them outright.

How children behave when they are admitted to the hospital varies widely. Anna Freud and her collaborator described the different types of children and their coping mechanisms in great detail (Bergmann and Freud 1972). Many children react to the situation by screaming, crying, or becoming aggressive, fighting fiercely against all the proceedings, including attempts to provide comfort. They often cause hospital staff substantial difficulties at the beginning, and a lot of patience is needed to deal with these children. As time goes on, however, these same children often develop into the patients who are most willing to accept medical assistance and the constraints imposed on them, "as if the uninhibited purging of fear, despair, and fury at the beginning had freed them, putting them in a position to use positive methods to master their situation."

Their opposites are the so-called perfect patients who seem to adjust serenely to the circumstances and whose conduct is cheerful and even considerate. These children probably do not dare confront the overwhelming feelings evoked by the situation. They expend all their energy fighting off fantasies that generate fear and anxiety. It is primarily these children who react later with behavioral disorders such as bedwetting or problems in school.

I have touched on only two behavior patterns at opposite ends of the scale, and not every child can be subsumed into one category or the other. But caregivers should be aware that a child who causes no difficulties at the beginning may be more likely to bring home problems resulting from their hospital stay without having worked through them than children who react strongly at the beginning and are able to give free rein to their rage.

A third group whose behavior I have observed with pleasure again and again are children whose parents have, from the very beginning, provided them security in a world in which they can feel safe. It is exciting to watch how these children, who are being admitted to a hospital ward for the first time, adjust to this situation. It isn't abnormal for children to cling to the coattails of the people accompanying them and from there observe the new surroundings with trepidation. But there are children who go exploring after a short time and even lose sight of their parents once in a while. We can assume that these children will have fewer difficulties surmounting the problems associated with their illness successfully. This is because they can depend on their parents not to leave them in the lurch, even in the most difficult of situations. So it doesn't frighten them to wander temporarily out of sight. Petrillo and Sanger (1980) studied the concerns of children who have to be admitted to the hospital as inpatients. They describe the following concerns:

- physical defects
- the extent of the illness
- impending or actual hospital admittance
- time spent with unfamiliar people

- difficulties in social interactions with family and friends
- the possibility of painful procedures
- hospital admittance as result of personal guilt or guilt on the part of parents
- unfamiliar routines and surroundings
- parental adjustment to new feelings of helplessness
- the need for independence
- the necessity of dealing with doctors and nurses

The concerns of affected adults are probably not so different.

Next I investigate the consequences of a hospital stay or a severe illness for children in different age groups, although in every age group an illness can have somewhat different consequences depending on the developmental stage of the child.

An infant must first develop the insight that it is autonomous and separate from others. This developmental process can be changed or interrupted by a serious illness. Forced changes in eating and sleeping habits, pain caused by various procedures, separation from the mother—a stay in the hospital can cause all this and more. An infant's inability to understand this context and the psychological and emotional traumas it causes can severely impair development at this age. This is particularly true when children's mobility and the associated possibilities for movement and learning through play are limited. That is why visual and auditory stimulation is important at this age, even if the child is seriously ill. Cribs should be strictly a place for resting, and no procedures of any kind should be carried out there. And parents should be encouraged to hold the baby in their arms as often as they can, even if they are limited by the monitor wires or tubes connected to body cavities. It is no doubt hard on parents not to be able to explain the situation adequately to their infant, but they are definitely in a position to calm and comfort the child. The baby feels the closeness and affection of a familiar person and depends on it.

Toddlers have reached a stage when they must develop autonomy and self-control. Pain, separation from their parents, and fears triggered by the unusual situation are likely to set off problems at this point; however, there is no fear of death as yet. Toddlers will react to the fears, depression, and sadness of parents in kind; they may also experience physiological or emotional regression. They lose recently acquired capabilities, and this frightens them.

Parents usually can't be as consistent with a severely ill child as they once were. But with no limits, toddlers feel insecure; we see this in healthy children as well, when parents fail to set limits. Parents should be encouraged not to change their consistent approach, even though it may be difficult. It is even more difficult if parents have to act consistently for the first time.

Young children, like children of all ages, need to be able to express themselves nonverbally. By engaging in creative activities like painting, making things with their hands, or singing, children can take constructive action even if the healthy part of their life has been disrupted. This way, children can create their own artistic symbols to express their fears. This applies even to toddlers (Gibbons 2001).

Walking, talking, control of bodily functions, and ability to be separated from their mothers are the important capabilities preschool children must develop. At this age, children immediately perceive painful therapies, separation from the mother, isolation, and immobilization as punishment for real or imagined misbehavior. As a result, the children regress, become aggressive, withdraw, or resume bedwetting. Uncooperative behavior and problems with sleeping are frequent. Nightmares are common at this age, and it is extremely important for the child to be able to express fears and worries. Telling stories that touch on illness and even indirectly on dying (for example, the death of animals) is one way for children to express themselves that is not anxiety-producing. At this age, children also clearly demonstrate their apprehension through roleplaying. It makes preschool children insecure if their parents' behavior obviously changes and they cease setting clear limits. Explanations are imperative, keeping in mind that children have no clear concept of time at this age. We have to make it clear to parents that children will understand if we tell them they have to sleep in the hospital again, but they cannot clearly understand concepts like or "tomorrow," much less "day after tomorrow."

School-aged children have developed a certain independence and autonomy. They concentrate on specific activities and are increasingly able to think through complex events. They feel increasingly able to assume responsibility, and in this way they gain self-esteem. If a hospital stay repeatedly interferes with the autonomy they have already established, feelings of incompetence and inferiority can develop. Children listen closely at this age, but they don't always understand everything they hear. So it is important to find out what the child knows and what he or she has really understood. School-aged children often don't ask questions, because they think everyone expects them to know a lot. At this age, open communication is indispensable. Unstructured play is still important, if for no other reason than because play makes it possible to forget the illness and all its problems temporarily. It is also important for us to assure children in this age group that their serious illness was not caused by inappropriate behavior.

Adolescence is definitely the most difficult age. The illness comes at that unfortunate point in time when adolescents question their own identity, want to become increasingly independent, and are particularly sensitive. Peer group acceptance plays a big role, and any physical impairment or disfiguration (severe acne or hair loss, for example) endangers security within the group and self-confidence. It is generally assumed that adolescence is a unified stage of development, but there are actually three quite different periods. An eleven-year-old boy sees things very differently from a nineteen-year-old (Gibbon 2001).

Early adolescence is determined by the beginning of puberty, when the body clearly changes. Increasing awareness of sexuality leads to insecurity with regard to the opposite sex. Authority is questioned, and friendships acquire a central role; their loss is experienced as severe. During this stage of life, a person is especially vulnerable. An awareness of the loss of childhood develops, as does fear of other changes.

Everything that characterizes early adolescence is also true of middle adolescence; indeed, some aspects are intensified. The parents' authority is fundamentally questioned. Independence from them is an important developmental goal during this time. This development is dramatically interrupted or at least temporarily brought to a halt by the illness, a situation that is hard for the young person to tolerate. Cognitive abilities develop impressively, but adolescents still don't think about the consequences of their actions. Their feeling of invulnerability can be prevalent at this age, which explains the typical readiness to take risks. This sense of immortality makes it especially difficult to confront illness and death, although adolescents are capable of doing so, especially if they themselves are affected. Although they certainly may think about the future, they live more in the present. The peer group is now more important than ever.

During late adolescence, young people become increasingly oriented toward the future. Their capability for abstract thought is fully developed, and feelings of inferiority are now based on a realistic self-assessment. At this age, an adolescent sees clearly what he or she will lose due to the illness. Parents gain in importance at this age. Sexuality has developed further, and often adolescents have entered serious partnerships, which are now threatened. This is an example of how the illness can force young people to abandon roles they have already assumed.

During the entire period of adolescence, humans develop independence yet are simultaneously dependent on the support of adults. Those who are healthy can decide the extent to which they want to ask for and accept help from adults, but adolescents who are ill are forced to accept the renewed dependency triggered by their illness. This, in conjunction with the loss of privacy that accompanies illness, can be catastrophic for young people. On the one hand, the result can be rage and aggression culminating in open hostility and refusal of therapy. On the other hand, adolescents increasingly think about the consequences of the illness for themselves and their families.

Everyone who is ill, and adolescents in particular, need options for distancing themselves from their illness, at least for a short time. Leisure time and vacations with family or fellow sufferers are helpful and invigorating. Adolescents can be a great help to each other, and inclusion in a group can provide tremendous security. But other adolescents may be overwhelmed if asked to provide help. This is especially true of established relationships. Sometimes the healthy partner feels caught in a web they cannot escape; everyone expects them to stand by their sick partner, and they expect it of themselves. Both partners in a situation like this urgently need support.

As mentioned earlier, hospital stays are usually associated with numerous procedures that are painful (drawing blood), cause anxiety (X-rays or MRIs), or require anesthesia (extensive examinations or operations). All children and adolescents, independent of age, have these feelings. We should prepare children as well as we can for what will happen to them. In addition, one parent should be present at an examination or accompany the child to the operating room. Many hospitals still require parents to leave their child at the operating room door; children often don't fall asleep until they are inside, and parents are not permitted to be with them at this moment. Anesthesiologists should be aware that they are making it unnecessarily hard on the children. There is really no reason for this practice except perhaps their own insecurity about having worried parents watching them during the induction of anesthesia.

Doctors are often told that children are hard to control and more likely to resist procedures if a parent is present. This is true in individual cases, and it sometimes takes patience to convince children of the need for a procedure.

And in individual cases, it may be necessary to send the parents out of the room in order to carry out the procedure without too much force. We have to remember that some children need to demonstrate their fear, their anger, and their helplessness to their parents. Some parents are frightened themselves and are not able to convey a sense of security to their children on a routine basis. It is often these children who have unusual difficulty with the procedures. To prevent parents from transmitting their own fears to their children, we must keep them well informed about what is happening to their child. And sometimes we as doctors have to have more patience with the parents of sick children than with the children themselves. It is impressive how often children will cooperate after initial difficulties if we employ enough patience and persuasiveness. It is true that we have to invest a lot of time at the beginning of treatment in order to win the trust of the children and their parents. This additional expenditure of time certainly seems problematic in a health care system that increasingly standardizes treatment procedures based on time. The expenditure of time is almost always worthwhile, however, and pays off later during the many necessary procedures. Some children, having already had bad experiences with doctors and hospitals, may therefore be fearful of what is to come.

Everyone who deals with children realizes that separation from the mother is a problem for them. This has been clearly verified in various studies (Freud 1943; Stern 1957; Spitz 1965). It would be a mistake to trivialize this issue, but by working together with parents, we can do a lot to minimize the trauma. If a toddler has to stay in the hospital for only a night or two due to an acute condition, we should do everything possible to enable one parent to remain overnight with the child. In the case of children who have to be inpatients multiple times or for a longer stay, on the other hand, it is appropriate to encourage parents to sleep somewhere other than the hospital. They desperately need sleep, and the hospital by its very nature is not a place where rest can be ensured. Many children understand this, and they also understand that their healthy siblings need a mother too.

That is why we should not give in too quickly to children's almost reflexive demand that mother and father be constantly present, even though we understand how they feel. When the hospital stay is lengthy, as it often is during therapy for malignant diseases, for example, it is important for the mother or father to catch their breath and recuperate. It is extremely tiring to keep infants and toddlers—or even school-aged children—in a good mood all day long under hospital conditions. Doctors or caregivers need to make this clear to parents and also to tell them that they won't be viewed as bad parents if they withdraw for a few hours to get some rest. Often parents have a guilty conscience, or they think they owe it to their sick child to be at the hospital around the clock, or they think that's what the treatment team expects.

Older children are definitely better at handling the contingencies of a hospital stay. When they are ill, however, they usually depend more than usual on their mother, and we cannot expect them to immediately recognize the logic of what is happening around them. A child may interpret the fact that his or her mother has placed him or her in a hospital as a sign that her love has decreased, even to the point that she wants to get rid of the child. Children often assume the blame for this supposed withdrawal of love, so they view the hospital stay as punishment. What child cannot find things in his past that he did wrong or for which his parents scolded him? Children with severe illnesses are the most likely to fear punishment, since they are desperately seeking the reasons for the incomprehensible things happening in their lives.

The hospital itself provides the child with plenty of cause for anxiety. Everyone needs time to adjust to new surroundings, and this is especially true of children. It is a well-known phenomenon that children don't like moving to a new town, even if nothing about their family situation will change. A change of environment is anxiety-producing for many adults, and this is even more true for children. The hospital often confronts the child with strange circumstances that can be extraordinarily frightening. Although we are trying much harder than in the past to create a child-friendly atmosphere in children's hospitals, the technical equipment cannot be concealed.

A lot has changed in recent decades, and many factors that used to instill fear in children have largely disappeared in the meantime. I have already mentioned that parents are present, often around the clock. The installation of playrooms with appropriate caregivers and of hospital schools has also made the hospital stay less monotonous for those children who are not too impaired by their illness. Today many children, even younger ones, have access to their father's or mother's laptop and are well versed in its use. Many hospitals now provide children access to the internet. This way they can stay continuously in contact with their siblings, their classmates, and their friends, an important thing for most children. Today's hospitals have integrated a substantial part of "normal" life into their routines, which clearly makes it easier for children and adolescents to adjust to the unfamiliar situation.

Very few research studies have dealt with children's concepts of their illnesses. One study treats the concepts of chronically ill children (Brewster 1982). Brewster assumed that chronically ill children learn a lot about their illness and for all practical purposes undergo an appropriate training program. Therefore it is important to understand what concepts children have in relation to their age. Brewster studied fifty children between the ages of five and thirteen who were hospitalized due to a chronic illness. She used the developmental concepts described by Piaget (1957, 1978) as the basis for her research. Individual results cannot be described here, but here are the conclusions Brewster drew from them.

- Caregivers must find out what the child understands and suit the explanations to the child's stage of development. Brewster cited Kohlberg (1963), who asserted that children can understand explanations tailored to the next developmental stage. She confirms this but did not view it as desirable in every case, since children should not be forced into a higher level of understanding.
- Brewster had the impression that well-informed children don't necessarily deal with their illness any better. In her opinion, temperament, the severity of the illness, and the family's coping style are better factors for predicting how children deal with illness. The greatest help for children who have difficulty is probably a change in behavior within the family that takes the new situation into account.
- Members of the treatment team must be careful that the kind of information they provide is not calculated merely to help them cope with their own frustration and helplessness.
- Children's magical thinking and their egocentric feelings are often defense mechanisms. We should be wary of puncturing them.

These interesting conclusions clearly show the influence of Piaget's concepts, as I discuss later. They also communicate important information for interacting with chronically ill children.

Despite our best efforts, the hospital is full of things that instill fear in patients. Even the context of normal and generally harmless occurrences is not transparent at first. The children have to deal with many unfamiliar people. Even today there are unfortunately still some staff in hospitals who are not friendly and have not understood how essential friendliness is in dealing with people who need help. This is also true for adult patients, of course. Children also feel the need to understand the treatment team's organization, and they may question individual team members about their roles. In addition, they become insecure and timid because they fear the effects of their illness and what is in store for them. Fortunately, children often dare to ask their questions and express their doubts, but they soon fall silent if it is made clear to them that such subjects are none of their business. It is impressive how even young children can handle the hospital situation after a short time if they perceive that people are open with them and are trying to help them with their problems.

CHAPTER FOUR

Children and Doctors

Being ill always means being dependent on others for help. The sick person is forced into a passive role. This is true of adults, and it is just as true of children and adolescents, of course. Children up to a certain age, however, are used to asking for help from adults and getting it, so for them the rupture in autonomy caused by the illness is not so severe. But when they reach adolescence, young people try harder and harder to free themselves from their dependence on adults. So they perceive the illness as exceptionally restrictive; after all, it sets them back to a stage they hoped they had at least partially left behind. Every doctor responsible for the care of children and adolescents must keep this in mind.

Numerous publications have clearly shown the doctor's essential function in the healing process; the patient's trust in him or her plays the primary role (see, for example, Bergmann and Freud 1972). Erich Stern (1957) summarized his thoughts on the matter as follows:

As we know, Freud characterized "transference" as the central problem in the doctor-patient relationship. The patient transfers the feelings and attitudes he had as a child for his father and mother to the doctor; he acts them out in inter-actions with him. In this regard, children and adults differ to some extent. For an adult, the father-child relationship belongs to the past; for a child, it is still in the present to some extent. We say "to some extent" because the phase in which parent-child relationships are formed, the so-called Oedipal phase, is already in the past for an older child. But inside him, it continues to have its effect, though in a completely different way, and the emotions and conflicts that were present earlier reappear in daily interactions with parents. It is still true that the doctor takes the father's place, and the child's behavior toward him is largely deter-mined by how he viewed and views his biological father, or to what extent the doctor resembles the father and assumes the paternal role. The child who trusts his father will usually also trust the doctor, or a teacher for that matter. The op-position the child may show, the rejection, hate, or fear he may express from time to time are not actually directed at the doctor, but at his father. This is only true in very general terms because the child's behavior will be considerably in-fluenced by the concrete role the doctor plays, by the task he has to accomplish, and by his entire personality. The ease with which the doctor gets to know the child is very important. It involves enjoying contact with children, an absolute requirement for a good pediatrician.

I quote Stern so extensively because on the one hand, he subscribed strongly to the psychoanalytic view of the role of the doctor—a man who oc-cupies the father's place. On the other hand, he made it clear that children's behavior toward a doctor is very much shaped by how parents and children interact with each other. Parents' reaction to their children's behavior is just as significant as the sense of security the children get from their parents. To put it the other way around, what's important is how consistently the child has felt that he or she could depend on his or her parents. This dependability is essential for developing the self-confidence the child will urgently need when external circumstances call everything they have thus far experienced into question.

Stern also discussed the mother's importance (a female attachment figure) in such circumstances, but he concentrated mainly on the male doctor, whom he placed at the center of his deliberations, as was typical during Freud's time and well into the second half of the twentieth century. Today more than half of pediatricians are women, so we could actually file away Stern's text as out-moded. Children do behave differently with male and female doctors. With a female doctor, they often behave as they would with their mother. Stern, however, was interested in the relationship between the child and both parents, not just between child and father. That children usually differentiate between male and female members of the treatment team is clearly demonstrated in their interactions with the nurses. Female caregivers often behave much like a mother; they are much more affectionate with the children, for example.

Children from Turkish families are especially likely to behave differently toward male and female doctors. Traditionally, boys take on a certain "pasha role" from their fathers that they adopt toward their own mother as well. The mother consents to this role, and the rest of the family accepts and sanctions it. As a result, boys are demanding in their behavior toward their mothers in everyday life, accepting their authority only in a limited way or not at all. They adopt this attitude toward the female members of the treatment team, too, whether they are doctors or nurses, making it hard for the boys to accept the influential and even dominant role of these women. This isn't specific to Turkish boys, of course; the same dynamic can be observed in children from other ethnic and cultural backgrounds. Often it is true for only children of single mothers as well, since male children must often substitute for the missing partner. They are cast in a role they cannot adequately play but that does give them limited or even pronounced dominance with respect to their mothers. So we can see how much children are shaped by their parents' behavior and by interactions with them, as well as by how they understand their own role based on the circumstances in their family.

Often doctors cannot avoid causing children pain—when drawing blood, for example—but giving advance notice sometimes makes such procedures easier to tolerate. Painful procedures usually cause infants nothing more than general feelings of displeasure, leading to a variety of reactions. Authors in the field of psychoanalysis agree that for toddlers, the experience of physical pain is linked to psychological perceptions (fears) that can set off corresponding reactions if repeated (Freud 1971). Anna Freud believed that "the psychological importance of the experience of pain explains why many children not only fear the doctor (and other people who have to cause them pain) but also love them. The experience of pain appeals to passive-masochistic impulses that play a large role in children's love lives. The child's bond to the doctor or nurse is often especially strong on the day after a painful medical procedure." This point of view is strongly influenced by psychoanalytic thinking, but we notice that children often don't seem to hold these procedures against the doctor. It may also be true that even relatively young children quickly comprehend that the doctor wants to help them and fight the illness, even though painful or at least unpleasant procedures may be necessary.

If children have never had limits set for them, or if they accept only limits set by their fathers, this will be clearly reflected in their behavior in the hospital. As they experience the routine of diagnostic or therapeutic procedures, they will soon perceive that many things don't and can't go the way they would like. Accepting this is especially difficult if they have never been in a comparable situation. The doctors in particular, but nursing staff too, must insist that children observe the established rules in their own self-interest. With this goal in mind, hospital staff need to have a lot of patience with the sick child. But if his or her cooperation can't be gained even with the greatest possible patience and powers of persuasion, we simply have to put our foot down. That can be traumatic for children who have never experienced anything like that before.

If the speed with which the disease progresses permits, it is always worthwhile to do everything possible to convince the child that the measures being taken are necessary. This way we can often lay a sound foundation for a future relationship right at the beginning of care. The situation is especially difficult if we are forced to take measures quickly in the sick child's own interest. It may be especially hard for children to accept the necessity for subsequent measures and to come to terms with the complex situations in which they find themselves over and over again in the course of treatment.

For doctors, winning a child's trust is crucial. To start with, children have to understand that they are now dependent on this new and unfamiliar adult. They need to learn as quickly as possible that they can depend on the doctor and that he or she will not lie to them. A doctor can say only once with impunity that the needle used for taking a blood sample won't hurt, because the needle does hurt and it will be obvious right away that he or she lied. How is the child supposed to know that this discrepancy won't always occur or may occur only occasionally and unpredictably?

Doctors have to be aware that not every child will like them right away. Many doctors, however, have trouble understanding this, don't consider the problem at all, or assume that members of their profession are intrinsically likeable. After all, if we are honest with ourselves, we have to admit that not every personality type appeals to us. This applies to everyone, whether doctor or patient. So it is better for all children (and all patients) if a doctor they have learned to trust carries out unpleasant procedures. It explains why it is both necessary and proper to allow children to express such preferences and to honor them whenever possible. Of course it hurts our feelings when we as doctors expend a lot of effort with a sick child only to have him or her prefer another doctor.

In the interest of their patients, all doctors, especially doctors who want to interact with children, have to develop the self-confidence to accept these preferences. If we allow children to decide in favor of a particular doctor, even "difficult" children often become much more cooperative. Children quickly grasp which doctor on the team is the most experienced. But they may choose to have blood drawn by an inexperienced beginner whom they like; this doctor may even be allowed a failed attempt or two without protest. This example makes it clear how helpful it is when the patient trusts the doctor as a person.

It is absolutely necessary to gain the trust of a seriously ill child at the outset, because it lays a good foundation for interactions throughout the course of treatment. This trust is especially necessary if all therapeutic efforts are useless and the child is dying. That is when a child most needs a doctor he or she trusts.

Whenever possible, doctors should avoid carrying out unpleasant examinations or procedures in the child's bed; otherwise they run the risk that the child will be frightened every time the door is opened. It is much better if children are brought to an examination room for every procedure. The presence of other people such as students is stressful for many children at first and may cause them to be less cooperative or even uncooperative. Observers may have to be asked to leave the room. Experience shows, however, that there is no major problem if the children have already gotten to know the students. We should still remember that many children and adolescents, especially older ones, feel they are being put on display. This is even more true when we want to present the child to a larger group of students or even to a class in a lecture hall. It has happened to me more than once that a child agreed at first but, upon seeing the many people in the seats, did an about-face and left me standing there without a patient to present. It has also happened to me that a child was willing to try a second time because he felt sorry about leaving me in the lurch and then quite bravely accompanied me.

In closing, I quote Stern once again, who commented that "there is no such thing as an attitude toward doctors per se, but there is always an attitude

toward a particular doctor, and everything depends on how the doctor re-
sponds to the child or adolescent." It is often harder to gain the trust of an
adolescent patient; it's possible that he or she has already had a bad experience. So adolescents are a particular challenge for doctors, one they must face
in order to practice their profession competently for their patients' benefit.

CHAPTER FIVE

Death and Dying in the Everyday Lives of Children

Before I discuss death and dying in the everyday lives of children, I would like to outline briefly how society in general deals with death, and how attitudes and behaviors have changed over time. A detailed description is beyond the scope of this chapter and would provide material for an entire book. For those who would like more information, I recommend the excellent books by Philippe Ariès (1976, 1980). In the chapter "Death Denied," he described how at the beginning of the twentieth century throughout the Western world, a death affected society as a whole, and the collective reaction was to keep the dying person involved in everyday life until the end (Ariès 1980). This is illustrated by Gottfried Keller's *The Governor of Greifensee,* mentioned in the introduction (1972). Dying usually took place at home, and at least the closest relatives were present so that everyone could say goodbye. Friends and acquaintances came too, and—at least in the Catholic Church—the priest appeared at the dying person's home accompanied by an acolyte in his vestments to perform the last rites, with bells ringing, in front of the whole community. So death occurred in full public view, not in secret.

In the second half of the nineteenth century, a dramatic change took place in the relationship between the dying person and his or her surroundings. As Ariès wrote, "Of course the discovery that his end was approaching was an unpleasant moment for every person. But people learned to cope with it. The church was keeping watch, and imposed on the doctor the obligation to play the messenger of death, the nuntius mortis. This was not a pleasant mission, and thus the efforts of the 'spiritual friend' were often needed for success in cases where the 'physical friend' still hesitated. If the advance warning didn't happen spontaneously, there were established conventions in the traditional customs of the church, such as, for example, the last rites."

The situation became more and more problematic around the start of the twentieth century, when what Ariès called the "beginning of the lie" developed. The sick person and the community around him put on an act for each other, a comedy intended to convey the message that "nothing has changed" or "life goes on as usual." Everyone got used to the charade. This had the practical advantage of removing or suppressing any signs that might alarm the sick person, in particular the staging of the public ceremony that began with the entrance of the priest. Even practicing Catholic families became accustomed to not calling the priest until his appearance could no longer make an impression on the dying person, because he or she was either unconscious or already dead. Thus the last rites became a sacrament for the dead and not for the dying, as originally intended. At the Second Vatican Council, the Catholic Church drew the obvious conclusion and replaced the last rites with the sacrament of the anointing of the sick, which is not administered solely to the terminally ill. With this change, the sacrament no longer functions as immediate preparation for death. Thus the church has admitted that it has no place in what happens at the moment of death and that there is no point in calling a priest at that late stage.

I have experienced how the administration of the last rites can frighten a dying person who is not prepared for it. I still remember a nineteen-year-old girl with cancer who first realized how close to death she was when a priest bearing the Eucharist arrived at her bedside in a solemn procession led by an altar boy ringing his bell. In this case the priest really had assumed the role of the nuntius mortis (the messenger of death) with his plan to administer the sacrament, for which none of the doctors had prepared the dying girl. I will never forget her horrified face as it dawned on her what the ringing of the bell meant. This approach to making the situation clear is harsh and unacceptable.

A new development began in the 1930s, leading to what Ariès called "hidden death in the hospital" (1980). The dying person's bedroom in the home, which had become an increasingly uncomfortable place for family members, was banished to the hospital. The increasingly technological nature of medicine and the advent of many sophisticated treatments available only in hospitals certainly contributed to this trend. So the hospital became the place where death, an unseemly event, ran its secret course hidden from the public eye. For the same reason it also became the place for a lonely death. In the meantime, the hospital has been increasingly replaced by the so-called hospice, a hospital to which the sick person is transferred for the process of dying. Without a doubt, palliative care is handled more professionally there both in terms of adequate pain therapy and emotional support. But it isn't as clear that death loses its "secret" character in this context, since here too it occurs behind closed doors. Family members can now be with the dying person here as they can in the hospital, but this represents only a faint reflection of an earlier way of thinking. It is hard to imagine that we will ever return to the public interaction with death typical of past centuries.

Children and adolescents are not excepted from this societal development, which has taken place in a similar way throughout the Western world. But it is not clear to what extent death in the public eye was also true for children. The Puritans in seventeenth- and eighteenth-century New England did tell children when death was impending (Stannard 1975; Slater 1977; Joy 1981). All children were encouraged to think about their own death, and this was especially true for sick children, who were prepared for the end of earthly existence this way. Death was not concealed from children in other countries either, as Keller (1972) described in *The Governor of Greifensee*. In the nineteenth century, death still wasn't hidden from children, but it was increasingly prettified (Pernick 1983). It was clear to the Puritans that death as punishment could strike whole communities including children, but the death of children was glorified in other places, as we see in nineteenth-century English literature, for example (Banerjee 1996). In the twentieth century, death acquired a secretive quality for children and adolescents too; the lie found its way in, and adults fell silent. This is one of the main subjects of this book.

The process of dealing with grief has also changed substantially. Earlier it was seen as appropriate to show grief and pain at a loss in public, as it is today in Greece or Islamic countries, for example; today in Western culture, this is no longer desirable. Today in our hospitals we hear the loud laments of members of Muslim families whose children have died, reminding us of the professional mourners of earlier times. The visit of condolence has been a thing of the past for a long time, and we are often asked to avoid expressions of sympathy at the graveside. Mourning has lost its public quality and has been declared a private matter.

Gorer (1965) defined three categories of mourners who have lost someone dear to them:

- There are people who repress the death and who prefer to deal with everything on their own. They force themselves to act as if nothing had happened. This attitude is not without its problems, and it inhibits the necessary coming to terms with grief.
- The second group discloses a little of their despair, so it isn't completely hidden from those surrounding them. Others are expected to notice the grief but not to feel too burdened or involved in it. In the final analysis, mourning remains a private matter. That is the behavior expected in our society. We accept that people who have suffered a loss caused by the death of a family member or friend will have an emotional reaction but without making excessive demands on third parties.
- Finally, there is a third group of the bereaved who display their grief openly over a long period of time. This is not welcome in our society; citing grief as a reason for declining an invitation to a party, for example, will often be met with a lack of understanding. People who display understanding for this behavior tend to be the exception.

We talk about the deceased as little as possible. This is a difficult problem, especially for the parents of children who have died, since the children are not allowed to live on, even in memory.

Children and adolescents often give loud expression to their anger about being seriously ill at the beginning, and it usually enables them to deal with it better in the long run. Lamenting and grieving aloud definitely have a similar positive effect. Yet we still have to accept that society doesn't want to change its way of dealing with grief. Ariès (1976) wrote: "It is obvious that the abolition of mourning is due not to the frivolity of the bereaved, but to cruel pressure from society. This society refuses to participate in the emotional shock of the ones who are suffering—thus negating the presence of death, even if it accepts death's reality in principle. . . . Today tears of grief are equated with the excreta of disease. Both are equally repellent. Death has been expatriated." This viewpoint is not changed by the fact that psychology views the repression of grief—correctly, I believe—as highly questionable. The general public has taken note of the discussions around death and care for the dying occurring in professional circles since the early 1990s; this is shown, for example, by the increasing interest in establishing hospices. The basic attitude described above has changed little, however.

Since the end of the nineteenth century, children and adolescents have been increasingly excluded from the process of coming to terms with the death of a family member or of an acquaintance. It is not very different today. We often do not take children along to a funeral. Their deceased grandfather has disappeared forever, and we rule out the possibility for them to come to terms with the new situation adequately. We don't want to burden the children, but with this approach, that is exactly what we do. We in the hospital have often experienced how sad the affected children become at being excluded, even though it was supposedly for their own protection. This is especially true if a person dies who is important to the child. Children should be allowed to participate in the funeral of such a person, even if their presence creates an additional burden because they need supervision.

After this general discussion of death in our society, it is time to look at the death of children. In Germany and other countries with few children, the death of a child is a special catastrophe. The same is true of a life-threatening illness that presupposes the loss of the child. It was not always this way. In preindustrial Western society, the death rate among infants and toddlers was high, and the death of children was part of everyday life. This is still true in many parts of the world, particularly in many African and Asian countries.

In Europe during the Middle Ages, fathers paid little attention to their newborn children. That did not change until their survival became more certain (Bürgin 1978). The frequency of infant death was a frustrating experience, and fathers shielded themselves from their feelings this way. People accepted a small child's death as they did the death of a young mother after a birth due to childbed fever. Otherwise, the death of a child, often followed quickly by the next one, would have been almost unbearable. Having several wives one after another was probably the only way to assure plenty of offspring. In many developing countries, such as the Central African Republic, this situation has not changed. Children there do not become individuals with their own rights until the age of six, and mourning for a deceased child has less to do with the loss of the child than with the loss of social prestige that often depends on the number of children (Bürgin 1978).

Well into the nineteenth century (and in developing countries today), the death of a sibling or another child was simply part of everyday life for children who survived beyond infancy or early childhood. This has changed in modern industrial society, and such an occurrence has become a rarity. Children today seldom need to cope with the death of a sibling, so death appears to have disappeared from their field of vision.

This does not mean, however, that children in our modern society are no longer confronted with death and dying. Rather the opposite is the case. Modern media, particularly television, present death in its various aspects, with accidents, war, environmental catastrophes, and death as a result of violence all figuring prominently. It is much less common for television to show children disease as the cause of death. Death was everpresent in nineteenth-century children's books, as we can see in many fairy tales or in *Struwwelpeter* (Hoffmann 1945). On the other hand, the portrayal of diseases and death in twentieth-century children's books played a minimal role for a long time. Probably the first author of children's books to pay attention to this topic was the Swedish writer Astrid Lindgren in her books *The Brothers Lionheart* (1995) and *Mio, My Son* (1998). Today the number of books for children and adolescents that deal with diseases and sometimes with death is much larger. Still, we cannot ignore the fact that television remains the most important source of information for children.

In the private sphere, on the other hand, death in Western society has largely been eliminated from the world of children. They seldom experience the death of a family member, of their grandmother or grandfather for example, which usually takes place in the hospital. They are seldom allowed to visit the sick person one last time, to say nothing of actually saying goodbye. If dying happens in the home, the children are often housed with another family to "spare them the upset." And they mustn't go to funerals either, since they will just be frightening for the children. Although adults are aware of the importance of saying goodbye within the framework of a funeral ritual, they usually don't acknowledge the same necessity for their children. As far as younger children are concerned, grandfather disappears mysteriously, and it's just a matter of time until he returns.

Children have to cope with society's divided attitude. This is anything but easy, and it's aggravated by the fact that adults avoid talking about death and dying because they have great difficulty with these topics themselves. A Swedish study showed that only one-third of the parents of children who were suffering from cancer and later died of it had discussed the topic at any time during their illness (Kreicbergs et al. 2004). Parents are usually convinced that their children are absolutely not interested, so they see little need to talk with them about it. This becomes a problem when it's no longer a matter of abstract concepts but of a real event in the family that vitally affects the child.

When children, especially preschool children, are playing, death and dying figure prominently in their games. Shooting the enemy is part of the ritual of roughhousing, and in their fury they sometimes send adults to Kingdom Come as well. Pretending to kill as a way of getting rid of aggression is often useful for a child. In *The Interpretation of Dreams,* Freud (1913) intensively examined children's hostility toward their siblings; the impulse is clearly expressed in children's dreams when they wish death on "rival and stronger playmates." Some sick children attempt to get rid of their anger at their serious illness by figuratively drowning or hanging their doctors and other members of the treatment team. They know perfectly well that this doesn't work, but it helps them control their anger. In all of these games and drawings, the children are aware that their activities won't have any serious consequences. Until they are about four, children don't perceive death as final. I discuss this point in more detail in chapter 8.

CHAPTER SIX

Physician Paternalism versus Patient Autonomy

Doctors in the West were in agreement until well after World War II that patients should rely unhesitatingly on the authority of the attending physician, an approach supposedly based on the tradition of Greek medicine in the ancient world. The patient is expected to believe that the doctor is more knowledgeable and will act in the patient's best interest. Galen, the Greek physician born in Pergamon in 129 A.D., said that the patient's trust is indispensable for the healing process. He also emphasized that this trust must be won through proper bedside conduct and thorough explanations as well as a mastery of prognosis (Porter 1997). It is clear that even nearly two thousand years ago, providing information to the patient was accorded an important role; medicine in the ancient world did not require the unconditional faith in the physician that doctors in the Western world during the modern period have generally expected from their patients. The majority of humankind had little idea what medicine could or could not accomplish. Medicine's ability to offer the sick person a cure was very limited as late as the second half of the nineteenth century, when rapid development of the natural sciences was accompanied by dramatic improvements in our understanding of the underlying causes of disease. Both doctors and patients were used to doctors' paternalistic attitude. Sick people had little reason to question this approach, and it established a relationship that was comfortable for doctors. The physician usually tried hard not to abuse this trust. Most people simply accepted occasional incidents of extremely authoritarian behavior toward patients; the famous Berlin surgeon Ferdinand Sauerbruch was reported to be an example, but he was widely considered to be a gifted doctor, so many sick people considered themselves lucky to be treated by him.

Several years after the end of World War II, it became public knowledge that atrocities had been committed by individual doctors in the concentration camps and that doctors were heavily involved in the politically supported destruction of "worthless life" and forced sterilization. For the first time, doubts about doctors' integrity were expressed openly (Mitscherlich and Mielke 1962).

After the Second World War, it became clear that it was not just a few misguided SS doctors who were involved in implementing the racist mania of the National Socialists in all its horrific aspects; respected members of the medical fraternity outside the concentration camps, in universities and hospitals for example, were also involved. They had voluntarily and actively submitted to the National Socialist ideology. Renowned scientists had participated in creating and representing the party's ideology of race. The medical profession seldom challenged the dehumanizing of groups such as Jews or gypsies. This "dehumanization" of some segments of the population in party propaganda gave many citizens an essential foundation for participating actively in the extermination of these groups or at least for condoning it. This was also, unfortunately, true of pediatrics as well; the Society for German Pediatrics (Gesellschaft der deutschen Kinderheilkunde) willingly expelled their Jewish members, who had made up more than 50 percent of the total membership (Seidler 2000).

As a result of revulsion on an international scale, and in particular as a reaction to the Doctors' Trial held in Nuremberg in 1946, committees of physicians developed codes of conduct intended to prevent a repeat occurrence of such cases (in 1948 the Declaration of Geneva and in 1949 the International Code of Medical Ethics, both from the General Assembly of the World Medical Association). An intensive discussion of the ethical behavior of doctors began. There was increasing awareness that physicians as a group could not be trusted unconditionally; this meant that patients could not unconditionally entrust their own care to every representative of the profession. The issue of so-called euthanasia did not begin with the National Socialists, however; its roots can be traced back much further. In 1896 in the United States, a eugenic movement in Connecticut led to a law that prohibited "epileptics" and "feeble-minded" people from marrying. This prohibition was later linked to a forced sterilization program to which over one hundred thousand people reportedly fell victim, so euthanasia was a subject of discussion in the United States by the end of the nineteenth century.

In 1920 Karl Binding, an expert in criminal law in Leipzig, and Alfred Hoche, a psychiatrist in Freiburg, published a short book sanctioning the extermination of life unworthy of life. Hoche held fundamentally the same opinions as the later National Socialists, since he denied the "personhood" of certain people. The National Socialists characterized the Jews as subhumans and later as vermin; for Hoche, it was the "incurably imbecilic" who were of "no value at all to either society or themselves as far as the continuation of life is concerned." Hoche himself wrote that "expressed in a more friendly way," these people have already suffered a "death of the mind," and someone who is already dead has no further right to life. In their book, both authors opposed the idea that doctors have a universal duty to extend the life of dying people who are suffering, and they advocated for the authorization of active help in dying, a position that is especially interesting from the perspective of today. This topic as it applies to children will be addressed in a later chapter.

After the Second World War, patients' rights increasingly became a focal point as a result of public debate. Damage suits against doctors contributed to this shift. In Germany, these trials were initially shaped by solidarity among doctors, who found it difficult to acknowledge a colleague's mistakes even when the mistakes were apparent to the judge. The result was a judicial "crutch" in the form of conviction due to failure to inform. As a prerequisite, the patient must be recognized as being of age and therefore able to request extensive information from his or her doctor about his or her illness and the planned diagnostic and therapeutic procedures. Failure to inform was declared an instance of medical malpractice in and of itself. Failure to inform about imminent death, of course, had no legal consequences; in this circumstance no plaintiff has yet brought forward a case. This development proceeded much faster in the United States than in Europe because of a system of justice that promised the patient ever higher damages.

In the framework of this examination of doctors' past and future conduct as well as the discussion of patients' rights, the paternalism that doctors had practiced for so long was abandoned, and the concept of the autonomous patient evolved. It would be beyond the scope of this book to describe this development in detail, but the context should be touched on briefly, since children as patients (and their parents) are subject to the system. Children have always been categorically denied the right to autonomy, and that is still largely the case today. From a legal viewpoint, they are not independent, and their parents have to make decisions on their behalf. So naturally children were not informed about what was going to happen to them. Legal practice ensured that parents had to consent to every intervention. To consent, they had to be sufficiently informed by the doctors. An intervention by a doctor without parental consent is still considered bodily harm.

In contrast, providing information to children is still not a legal issue, with the sole exception of the German Drug Law, which requires the consent of older children and adolescents, along with that of their parents, for participation in clinical trials. This topic, however, is being included more often in discussions of ethics. Getting consent in clinical drug trials (*consent* is the term used in Anglo-American texts) is being replaced in the case of children and adolescents by the term *assent,* which is intended to convey that researchers should obtain this group's agreement to their participation in the study. Both concepts are translated into German as *Zustimmung, Einwilligung, Billigung,* or *Genehmigung.* The Anglo-American literature makes a distinction, however, that can be described in our context as follows. Parents have to agree to children's participation in a clinical drug trial for legal reasons (consent); the children are simply asked whether they agree to take part to assure that they are not being forced to participate against their will (assent).

After the Second World War, paternalism was slowly replaced by the idea of patient autonomy in the medical treatment of adults. Autonomy in this case meant the sick person's freedom to decide whether to consent to the treatment suggested by the doctor or refuse it. Many doctors found this difficult; after all, they had to give up their dominant position and enter into a relationship with the patient that was virtually a partnership. An ethic based on responsibility (the doctor is responsible for decisions) was increasingly replaced by a contract-based ethic (the doctor explains various treatment options with their advantages and disadvantages and then leaves the final decision about how to proceed to the patient). In other words, the patient enters into a contract with the doctor regarding the mode of treatment.

If the doctor adheres strictly to this approach, patients often feel abandoned, left to deal with their problems alone. If these are critical decisions, perhaps even determining life or death, patients may feel overwhelmed, and the highly touted advantages of autonomy may become a burden. Providing complete information about potential (and rare) side effects of a medication or therapy as required by law, for example, can be extremely unsettling for the patient, particularly if the process is carried out solely to comply with legal regulations. In the meantime, many doctors have learned to handle the difficult situation created by the tension between patients' autonomy on the one hand and their helplessness on the other. If a good relationship has been established, doctors will be able to provide all the essential information to their patients without overwhelming them. It is much more important, however, to avoid leaving the sick person to make difficult decisions alone; instead, doctors should advise their patients and ultimately communicate their own views of the best possible treatment option. This is not a reversion to paternalism, because this approach lays a foundation the patient can use in making an autonomous decision. But it also enables patients to delegate responsibility either wholly or in part to the doctor they trust, a responsibility doctors must not shirk. An experience I had some time ago can serve to illustrate how important this responsibility is.

Later, I sometimes asked myself how I had come to take on the responsibility for this young woman who was not even my patient. She had not directly asked me to do it, nor had she expressly delegated it to me. But I had long ago learned from children that you have to read between the lines if you want to understand their wishes and perceptions. They don't always express what they want unambiguously, but they often send signals that we need to receive. I will not deny that a mistaken interpretation can have serious consequences, but fear of making a mistake should not be a reason for denying a sick person the help they need.

One could argue that this patient was an adult; what about children and adolescents? Can we and must we give these young people complete informa-

SEVERAL YEARS AGO I received a call from a colleague at another university who was a specialist in internal medicine. He asked me to advise a female patient for whom he was to perform a life-saving bone marrow transplant. She had asked permission to get a second opinion, and he promised to arrange a consultation. That was all he told me. I agreed, and a few days later his patient appeared at the scheduled appointment. The patient was a twenty-six-year-old doctor. An unusual blood count had been noticed during her pre-employment physical examination, and she was soon diagnosed with chronic myeloid leukemia. At that time a cure was possible only with a transplant, if an appropriate bone marrow donor was available. There was one in her case, because she had a brother, and the surface properties of his body cells were identical to hers. He was also prepared to act as donor. This type of leukemia has a distinctive feature that differentiates it from all other types of leukemia. The patient reported that she had no idea during the checkup that she might be sick. She felt fine, and the abnormal blood cell count surprised everyone.

Here is the problem the young woman was faced with. The so-called chronic phase of this type of leukemia can last for up to twelve years. Because the patients have no symptoms, it is often not possible to tell at the time of diagnosis how long the chronic initial phase has been going on. At some point, often without any recognizable symptoms, the disease progresses to acute leukemia. This form is not curable with medications, and only in a certain percentage of patients can therapy retard the progress of the disease. The longer the duration of the disease, the lower the success rate of the transplant. The young doctor was advised not to wait too long after the diagnosis to have the transplant; it should be scheduled within the next six to twelve months, and under no circumstances should she wait until the appearance of the acute phase. A transplant can still be done at that point, but the results are much worse. A wide range of statistics shows that without a transplant, 50 percent of chronic myeloid leukemia patients die within four and a half years. But a bone marrow transplant carries its own risk; depending on the stage of the illness and the hospital carrying out the procedure, 10 to 20 percent of patients die of the side effects of this life-threatening and stressful therapy. This gives a picture of the dilemma in which the patient found herself. Her husband, who was not a doctor, left the decision to her because he thought she had a much better understanding of the situation.

Continued

After we had gotten to know each other a bit and she had told me the history of her illness, she came to the real problem. She had given birth to a little daughter a year earlier, and she was thinking primarily of her daughter as she considered her options. It was obvious that she understood the peculiarities of her illness very well. She had visited the transplant center, where they had urged her to go ahead with a transplant. From a medical viewpoint, this recommendation was certainly technically correct. But the decision was obviously not quite so simple for her.

"If I don't go through with the transplant, my daughter might soon be without a mother, because my illness will kill me," she said. She continued, "But I may live another twelve years and my daughter will have her mother during her childhood." I just nodded; she didn't expect me to answer. "If I go through with the transplant, I may die of the side effects, and my daughter will lose her mother very quickly." She was silent for a moment and then continued, "But the transplant may also restore me to good health, and I would be here for my child for a long time to come." She had captured the dilemma in a few words. Then she looked at me and said, "I don't know what I should do."

The young woman sitting in my office was at her wit's end. She needed more than the advice of a specialist. She was not able to take responsibility for herself, and it was clear that she wanted to delegate it to me. Perhaps she hoped that a pediatrician could better understand her dilemma concerning her young daughter.

Like so many times in my life as a doctor, my objective was to come up with an adequate response in a reasonable amount of time. The thoughts were whirling around in my head. She had described the situation well; I didn't need to correct anything. Her husband wasn't ready to help her or didn't feel competent to make a decision for her or even to contribute to her decision. Should I get out of the situation by simply confirming that her oncologist and my colleagues at the transplant center were right? From both a legal and a medical viewpoint, this approach would be correct. But would that be helpful to her? She had not come to me simply to get a confirmation. I took the bull by the horns and said, "If you were my wife, I would proceed with the transplant." I still remember how hard it was for me to say this. Usually when parents in difficult situations ask me how I would decide if it were my child, I answer that I would leave the decision up to a doctor I trusted. How should I know what I would do if it were my own child who was seriously ill? But it wasn't the case that the young doctor didn't trust her colleagues. Nevertheless, she needed a decision, and she had obviously delegated that responsibility to me. So I undertook to make the decision for her. She looked at me for a moment, then nodded, stood up, thanked me in a few simple words, and left. I sat there for quite a while brooding. Had I done the right thing? Six months later I heard that her transplant had been successful and she had gone back to work. She hadn't thought it necessary to inform me. But that really wasn't important. She couldn't know that the matter had worried me for a long time; after all, after listening to my advice, she might have died as a result of the transplant.

tion and include them in decisionmaking? This is stipulated by law only in the limited circumstance described earlier, for the participation of children and adolescents in drug trials. In every other situation the parents alone have the right to decide. I believe that children who have reached a certain age and adolescents must be included in the fundamental decisions that affect them—termination of a cancer therapy, for example. It is not possible to specify a particular age; the doctor has to decide this for each child individually. There are five- and six-year-old children who can understand the issues of their case quite well. And after the age of eight, I think that most children can do so. The principle of autonomy is valid for them too. Of course we doctors have to think about how well each child is able to understand the context in order to make a meaningful decision. The children, and of course the parents too, have to live with the results. So we cannot exempt parents by taking away their legal responsibility, and this would usually not be in the children's interest either, since they want to have confidence in their parents.

But we should find out what children think and want, even if it sometimes conflicts with parents' wishes. We have no right to take away their autonomy, and neither do parents. The temptation is great; we know so much more, and we have the best intentions toward our patients. And we have more experience than our patients. One patient's story can show the potential effects of neglecting the principle of autonomy.

I tell this story here not to describe my poor conduct as a doctor, although it is important to recognize that it happened. I tell it to make it clear that a patient, even a child, can make an autonomous decision only if they receive

BERND WAS A thirteen-year-old boy with acute lymphoblastic leukemia. After his initially successful treatment, he suffered a relapse. A bone marrow transplant was his only chance of survival. He had an older brother who qualified as a donor and was willing to donate his bone marrow. His parents agreed to that course of action after I had given them the full information. We decided that I should talk with the boy and explain the situation to him. We were sure he would be happy that this possibility was available to him. The relapse had been a big shock because he had thought himself almost completely cured.

So I went to see him and explained the situation to him in detail. Bernd listened attentively. He asked hardly any questions, but it was obvious that he understood everything very well. I was about ready to end the conversation by saying that we would go ahead with the plan as I had described it when he suddenly said, "I don't want to. You can tell that to my parents." I must admit that I was shocked by this unexpected statement. I couldn't understand how he had come to this decision. I had explained everything clearly, and the situation was unambiguous based on the available evidence: he would die without a transplant. I had had enough experience with this therapeutic method and knew what I was suggesting. I had performed successful transplants on a substantial number of children and adolescents. And now this boy was saying that he didn't want to be saved. I can still remember that I was almost insulted. My intentions were good, and all the available data supported my view. In response to my pointed questions, he just shook his head and didn't answer. Finally he repeated his negative position without giving any reason for it and made it clear to me that he considered the conversation over.

I left, angry at him because he didn't want to believe me. I couldn't convince him that my intentions were good, and I was angry at myself and at the situation in which I found myself. Now I had to go to his parents and report my failure. His parents were appalled; they wanted everything done that was humanly possible to save their child. We agreed that we would not accept his negative response. We tried, both separately and together, to dissuade the boy from his "wrong" decision, and finally we succeeded. He agreed to the transplant. At first it went well, and inwardly I felt rather triumphant. But then a chronic rejection reaction set in, a much-feared immunological complication of bone marrow transplants. Despite every possible therapeutic effort, it grew steadily worse. Finally, after much suffering, the boy died.

I was dumbfounded. Did he oppose the transplant because he had a premonition of what would happen? Something like that might very well be possible. I can't say what the basis might be for such a premonition. But now I realize that the boy fought for his autonomy and lost the battle to us. In the end, he probably agreed to the transplant for his parents' sake because he understood how much they were suffering. He may have wanted to humor me too, since I had always treated him very well. I had done everything right from both a medical and a legal point of view. But as a human being, I had clearly failed. I resolved that in the future I would continue to try to convince my patients of the necessity for a particular treatment. But at the same time, I hoped I would never again try to talk a patient into a treatment.

information that is detailed and honest. This is widely accepted today for adult patients, but many doctors do not consider it valid for children and adolescents.

Parents have the right to insist that we do everything in our power to cure their children. Their fear of losing a child is boundless, and they hope, often against their better judgment, that it will not happen. So we can understand that it is hard for them to discontinue treatment, even in cases where it has long been clear that we have exhausted all the worthwhile treatment alternatives. Many parents find themselves in this dilemma: they want neither useless suffering nor an early death for their children. Without help, they often see no way out of this situation.

There is an extensive discussion taking place about when we should grant self-determination to children. Many children have acquired a lot of experience in the course of their severe illness, and age is not an unambiguous criterion. This is equally true with respect to their concepts of death, as we shall see. We need to find out in every individual case what children are thinking about and what they know. The younger the child, the more difficult this is. Many ethicists think a threshold is reached at age eight, and I have already emphasized that I believe most children can understand self-determination after age eight. I think it is actually better not to commit ourselves to a specific age, however, but to sound out the situation by talking with the children and their parents. The whole hospital team can help find out something about the child's ideas. Conversations with a nurse or other staff member may reveal aspects of the child's way of thinking that others don't know about. I cannot repeat often enough that children don't open up to just anyone. We adults don't do it either!

Each child, just like each adult, has a right to autonomy, and young children in particular convey their ideas nonverbally, through pictures and stories. They may delegate their decisions to us doctors or to their parents, as the young doctor whose story I told earlier did. If we begin with the general premise that children too have a right to make autonomous decisions and if we accept this premise as valid, then we will find it easier to understand that in particular instances children aren't able to make use of their autonomy; the child may be too young, the situation may be too difficult, or the child may not want to oppose his or her parents. Children always want to remain loyal to their parents. And they are prepared, as adults are also, to delegate responsibility for themselves. We doctors need to recognize this wish by talking with the children; otherwise we will not do justice to them and their ideas.

CHAPTER SEVEN

The "Precociously Mature" Child

All parents are convinced that their child is "something special." That view is understandable, and in general we can say that every human being per se is something special. Often enough, however, parents of seriously ill children overshoot the mark. They feel the need to emphasize, based on the child's life up to now, that he or she was always exceptional, especially when compared to siblings. Parents hope to make the listener understand how terrible it is for them that this child in particular may die.

If the loss of a child is potentially imminent—through a life-threatening illness, for example—the parents' instinctive reaction may be to idealize the child. This is not a problem as long as the parents' attitude doesn't give siblings the impression that their sick brother or sister is a first-class child and they themselves are second-class. But there is a great danger that they may come to this conclusion, especially if parents are constantly elaborating on the exceptional qualities of their sick child to anyone who will listen. We have to realize what it means for children when they feel their parents love them less than their siblings. A good example is the film *Walk the Line* (2005), which recounts the life of the country singer Johnny Cash. As a child, he experiences the death by a terrible accident of an older brother whom he loved and who was the apple of his father's eye. Instead of consoling Johnny, the father comes to the terrible conclusion that the devil had taken the wrong boy by mistake.

It is part of the caregivers' responsibility, be they doctors or psychologists, to make it clear to parents that their behavior threatens to have sustained aftereffects on the family. This is no easy task, since no one wants to take away the parents' conviction that their sick child is very special. Fortunately, asking questions about the qualities and characteristics of healthy siblings often shows parents quickly that they have several "special children" and that the sick child actually had no special status in the family *before* his or her illness. Only children are naturally something "special" for their parents or mother, particularly if they were born after a long period of childlessness or to an older mother at the end of her reproductive life. This situation is amplified if the father is not the mother's life partner; these children often take on the role of partner substitute. Of course, in these cases there are no other children who can feel disadvantaged by the parents' attitude.

There is also the idea that dying children are "people with a precocious spiritual maturity" (*früh seelisch vollendete Menschen*), as the well-known Viennese pediatrician Hans Asperger described children with leukemia in an article published in 1969. At that time, such children had no real chance of survival at the point of diagnosis. He had studied the behavior of sick children intensively, and one of my most impressive memories is of his introducing a sick child during a lecture, both because of the child's illness and because of his unique personality. Asperger seemed profoundly affected by the hopeless situation a leukemia diagnosis represented for a child at that time. The children were young for the most part, since the occurrence of acute lymphoblastic leukemia is highest during early childhood.

Asperger described these children as showing an unusual maturity in their personality development because of their illness. These sick children "had always been completely different from 'normal' children, who are vigorous, vivacious, easygoing, and good-humored; they are determined to assert themselves vis-à-vis parents and friends occasionally with anger and defiant behavior, sometimes with a 'touch of wickedness.' Children with leukemia are completely different. From an early age, they display an unusual subtlety in the realm of emotion; they have a delicate understanding of how others are feeling, and react with a profound kindness that is very unusual in someone so young."

He described how such a child has an unchildlike, mature piety not acquired, as is usually the case, from his or her parents, and he perceived a noticeably tragic underlying mood. He quoted from the *Duino Elegies* (1922) by Rainer Maria Rilke (who also died of leukemia), "For the beautiful is nothing more than the beginning of the terrible." Asperger speculated that "this constitutionally inherent delicacy may make these children susceptible to toxins that would not harm someone more robust." And he compared them with precocious artists like Mozart, Schubert, Egon Schiele, and Georg Trakl, all of whom worked frantically and recklessly wore themselves out in a short time. In 1942 a film was made about Wolfgang Amadeus Mozart; its title, *Those Whom the Gods Love,* would have to be continued with the assertion . . . *Die Young.*

Asperger closed his article as follows: "Perceptions like this help grief-stricken parents bear their pain more easily—and it is one of the noblest aspects of a doctor's work to serve as intermediaries for such perceptions. But the doctor, too, becomes more mature through experiences like this, becomes clearer about himself and his responsibilities, is forced to get his own life in order, is called even more strongly to feel loving sympathy with the sick person."

I quote Asperger so extensively because his statements are worth reading and sometimes to the point, but they are not unproblematic. Let's first look at the analogy he draws to the lives of artists who die young. He argued that precociously mature artists exhaust themselves physically through their intense creativity, to the point that they have little resistance to illnesses. The image of Mozart as one whom the gods love and therefore take at a young age dates from the Romantic period, when it seemed appropriate to put Mozart on an even higher pedestal by creating melancholy and sentimental biographical episodes such as the pauper's burial, the image of the unrecognized and starving artist, or death by poison. The image of the artist working so frantically that he "wears himself out" fits into this list. Reality looked very different in Mozart's case. For one thing, he was a successful artist, very famous in his own time, who earned well but didn't know how to manage money. For another, he probably died of an underlying disease, most likely recurring rheumatic fever, made more serious by the frequent bloodlettings, customary at the time, that were carried out by his doctor and progressively weakened him. The so-called pauper's burial with the collapsible coffin was based on a decree issued by Emperor Joseph II, who opposed the baroque pomp of the church.

If we look at the biographies of other artists, we see that many died at an advanced age; Johann Wolfgang von Goethe is an example. And as a counter-example to his own thesis, Asperger described the writer Theodor Fontane, who didn't begin writing his most important works until he was seventy, so clearly he had not worn himself out at an early age. I am convinced that we should abandon the image of early death as tied to precocious maturity in the case of particular individuals, as touching as it may be. It is simply the case that children who are forced to die young can neither complete their personal development nor attain a place in the adult world that would allow them to be involved in shaping the future. And there is no evidence that children with leukemia differ in any fundamental way from other children, as Asperger assumed. I have often heard parents say they can't understand how their child, so normal and always so healthy, can suddenly have become so seriously ill.

But what about Asperger's statement that idealizing a child who is sick with leukemia can help parents better endure their loss? Certainly it does accommodate the desire to understand the illness's cause and the loss connected to it; the actual cause of leukemia is unknown. But this approach might have the temporary or permanent effect of making it especially difficult for parents to endure the loss of their "unique" child. And the belief that God takes early those he loves most is hard to convey, even to devout Christians. It means that God's decision must be accepted with little protest.

Parents often ask doctors about their position on religious belief. If they do, experience demonstrates that it is helpful for believers in particular when doctors say they cannot understand why God would act in this way. And for many parents, it is an unbelievable relief when the hospital pastor shows understanding for their anger at this God who has incomprehensibly taken away their child. And if we as doctors promote parents' idealization of the dying child, it will have a lasting effect on the healthy siblings, who may have to live forever with the feeling that their parents were forced to surrender the best and most important child among them. These children, however, who have been downgraded to second-class status, might be able to perform an important function by making it easier for their parents to endure their loss. After all, these children, like their parents, live on.

It helps very little and may even be harmful if doctors convey to parents, or strengthen a conviction they already hold, that their dying child possesses a uniqueness worthy of being idealized. It tends to hinder them from working through their anger, rage, and despair, feelings that trouble almost all parents who lose a child. It is not a contradiction to say, however, that we need to talk with parents and siblings about what an important role the child who has died or is dying played in the family unit and for each individual, and how important it is for everyone that this person existed. Doctors, nurses, and other caregivers and members of the treatment team can convey to the parents that they are happy that they got to know the child. This is often true, because interacting with severely ill and dying children is not only a burden; it often provides beautiful and intense experiences that more than outweigh the worries and burdens.

I would have agreed with Asperger had he attributed a special and accelerated personality development to sick children. But he emphasized explicitly that it is a special sensitivity, either congenital or acquired in early childhood, that weakens the body's resistance to the outbreak of a serious illness. It is in fact impressive for caregivers to experience how quickly the personalities of severely ill children and adolescents develop and what a rapid maturation process they undergo during their illness. They have experiences because of their illness—loss of confidence in their own bodies or confrontations with death, for example—that accelerate the development of their personalities.

Many doctors assert that part of their uninhibited childhood is stolen by the illness. That is *one* way of looking at it. But we shouldn't forget that many events in a child's life can produce similar effects. A parents' divorce is surely much more traumatic for affected children than we are ready to admit in our divorce-happy society. Children's teachers also report again and again noticeable personality changes when former patients return to school after treatment. And the children themselves often view the behavior of their contemporaries as silly—when they get excited about things the children who have been ill view as unimportant, for example. And children and adolescents who have been ill often view school itself in a different light because they have given more intensive thought to their future.

Children do become "different" people because of their illness, and they look at life differently than their contemporaries. Their sensitivity to the problems and worries of others increases, and it will not come as a surprise that children who have faced a serious illness often go into one of the helping professions. Nevertheless, this fact should not mislead us into seeing the meaning of an illness in this development; a severe illness has no meaning in and of itself. At best, we can *give* it a meaning this way, and this sometimes helps make the consequences of the illness more bearable. In conclusion, I would emphasize that children who have faced a life-threatening illness are not "special" children per se, as Asperger believed, but illness does cause them to experience an unusual and accelerated development. And it helps parents if we discuss these aspects with them.

CHAPTER EIGHT

Healthy Children's Concepts of Death

Before we can answer the question of how children deal with death, we first need to clarify whether children think about death and dying at all. Some readers may be surprised that we ask such a question; after all, even young children deal with death in a playful way when they shoot each other and then drop to the ground, "fatally wounded." Often they lie there for a long time, motionless, and announce that they are now dead. That they soon get up again and continue playing, completely unaffected, is comforting for adults. It signals that the child isn't taking it very seriously. It is not as simple as that, however. The children's behavior does provide evidence that they don't view death as final in that moment, but does it prove that children don't think about death in any fundamental way, as has long been claimed? Even today, many adults, professionals such as doctors among them, like to assume that they do not. I do not intend to review all of the literature—some of it quite contradictory—on this topic; instead, I concentrate on some of the researchers' ideas that diverge in an elemental way.

Dieter Bürgin undertook an extensive critical review as early as 1978. It is true that his conclusions are not entirely in line with our ideas today. In the beginning, the fields of child psychiatry and child psychology paid little attention to the topics of death and dying. It was actually psychoanalysis that investigated this problem area as early as the first half of the twentieth century (Hug-Hellmuth 1912; Freud 1913, 1915a, 1915b; Deutsch 1919, 1937; Klein 1921, 1936; Bromberg 1933; Schilder 1934; Piaget 1978). Other disciplines, developmental psychology in particular, followed later (Bowlby et al. 1952; Piaget 1953; Childers and Wimmer 1971; Bürgin 1978; Candy-Gibbs et al. 1985). Examining the subject of death and dying is still not part of the educational program for younger children in Western society, even though they are confronted with it almost daily on television.

In her book *Weltwissen der Siebenjährigen* (The world-knowledge of the seven-year-old), Donata Elschenbroich describes what abilities and experiences we expect from seven-year-olds (Elschenbroich 2002). The broad spectrum covers capabilities and knowledge that many experts such as educators and developmental psychologists expect seven-year-olds to know or to have learned. Dealing with death is not among them. It would not be surprising if the spectrum included only facts and techniques. But she also mentions dreaming, knowing, and the reality that not all wishes can be fulfilled immediately. Even the topic of pregnancy and life before birth are included in a chapter entitled "Ich, ein Ankunftswesen: Die Monate und Wochen vor der Geburt—phantasiert, erinnert" ("Myself, an Arriving Being: The Months and Weeks before Birth—Fantasized, Remembered"). The topic of saying goodbye to life should, in my opinion, be included too. But in our society, the will to protect children as long as possible from that kind of knowledge is too pronounced.

Interest in children's death concepts appears very early in the literature of psychoanalysis and developmental psychology. Their fundamental concern is with children's ideas about their own death and dying, but they are also concerned with their ideas about the death and dying of familiar people. Such concepts are investigated within these two disciplines with their usual methods, including interviews, questionnaires, targeted observations, and drawings. A number of investigations led to attempts to identify age-specific concepts, since children's ideas depend on their age and their experiences. I introduced the term *death concepts* in this chapter for historical reasons, although I am actually less interested in structured concepts; they are always strongly influenced by the methodology of any given study and can only reflect the information it can encompass. But concepts are still important and necessary as a basis for further investigation. In the end, the way children think is far more complex than can be reflected in structured concepts.

In this section, I investigate what we know with relative certainty about how concepts of death develop in children. That most authors, predominantly developmental psychologists or educators, have studied only healthy children presents a major problem. Few authors deal with children who are dying or even sick. There are undoubtedly a wide variety of factors that influence the findings and even the investigations themselves. The children's own previous experiences definitely play an important role. The methods used sometimes differ greatly, which is also true of the types of children studied. The studies were carried out on very different groups of children (healthy children, children with noticeable psychological problems, children with somatic disorders, children who had lost close relatives, and children in a variety of age groups). Researchers also drew on adults' memories in order to be able to say something about how children think. And the methods used also have a substantial influence on the results (for example, structured or unstructured interviews, observations of play and behavior, interpretation of pictures, the use of projective tests).

Bürgin (1978) pointed out that the investigators, their mode of processing information, and their expectations are factors that play a major role with subject matter that is so fraught with emotion. It makes a big difference whether the investigator is statistically manipulating available data or working personally with the children. It also makes a difference whether healthy or sick children are being studied, although there are few studies in which this difference plays an important role; usually it is not even addressed. But conclusions about sick children extrapolated from studies of healthy children may be problematic. I return to this point at the end of the chapter. The question which interests us first, however, is how terminally ill children deal with death and dying and how they think about it.

The extent to which children are confronted with death in daily life is also an important factor. In preindustrial society, it was part of children's daily life to have little siblings who did not survive the first weeks or months of life. Older children were also threatened by infectious diseases against which there were no vaccines. And all of these situations still exist today in developing countries with high child mortality rates, particularly in the first year of life. Today we can scarcely imagine what it meant when a scarlet fever epidemic swept through the country and claimed the lives of several children in a school class or even from the same family. In the Dorotheenstadt Cemetery in Berlin, for example, you can find a family grave where four siblings are buried along with their parents, all having died from scarlet fever within a few weeks. And this was certainly nothing unusual.

Families didn't conceal the death of an adult just because there were children present. Death in the hospital, far removed from the person's own surroundings, as is typical in our modern society, did not yet exist. Instead, death occurred at home in one's own bed, usually with family members present. And children were not excluded from such events. We must admit that we don't know much about what children thought during this time. All the reports are from adults who later tried to remember what went on in their minds then—when their beloved grandmother died, for example. It's probable that their memories have been falsified or at least modified by later life experiences or interpretations so that their validity is rather limited. Memories are not much help in our effort to understand how children think, so I will not pursue this approach further. It is true that we know little about what children were thinking in the preindustrial period or at the beginning of the industrial age. It's worth reminding ourselves, though, that a positive evaluation of childhood and of the final phase of children's lives was an important theme in English novels of the Victorian period (Anthony 1940). And the episode from *The Governor of Greifensee* by Gottfried Keller (1972) cited in the introduction shows that at the end of the nineteenth century, people on the continent also considered children capable of dealing with death.

Concepts of death are not innate; they have to be acquired in the course of life. This is just as true for concepts of "life" (Cotton and Range 1990). And the two are intimately connected. Developmental psychologists agree that these concepts are dependent on age, maturity, and development—in particular the development of intelligence and of the sense of time. It is interesting to try to understand how representatives of various disciplines have investigated the development of children's concepts of death and what conclusions they reached. It was Sigmund Freud who first addressed this topic in *The Interpretation of Dreams* (1913). There he wrote about children's animosity toward their siblings, which is expressed in dreams about their death:

> Now perhaps someone will interject: "Granted the hostile impulse of children towards their siblings, but how could a tender infant disposition reach such heights of wickedness as to wish its rivals or sturdier playfellows dead, as if every

offence were only to be expiated by the death penalty?" Anyone who says this is not taking into account the child's idea of "being dead," which has only the word and very little else in common with ours. The child knows nothing of the horrors of decomposition, of freezing in the cold grave, of the terror of endless Nothingness which the adult's imagination cannot bear to contemplate, as all the myths of the world to come bear witness. The fear of death is unknown to the child; that is why he will play with the terrible word.

Then Freud explained his ideas about how children think: "To the child, who is, after all, spared the scenes of suffering before death, being dead is much the same as 'being away,' no longer disturbing the survivors. The child does not distinguish how this absence comes about, whether on account of a journey, an estrangement, or death."

Freud's choice of words is striking; it obviously reflects his own great fear of death, which must have troubled him at that time. It is interesting that Freud did not examine the relevant literature of the previous century (Keller's works included), which spoke in a clear but different language. We can see clearly, however—and this is much more important—that he categorically denied children the capacity to experience fear of death or have any understanding of death at all. This denial eliminates any necessity for adults to discuss death with children. This idea was doubtless a relief for him and lifted a burden from adults' shoulders. It had a decisive influence on the attitude of pediatricians into the last quarter of the twentieth century. And until the 1960s it went practically unquestioned.

Freud believed that children could not differentiate among different forms of absence. He was therefore certain that children had not yet acquired the concept of object permanence, which is necessary for understanding that being absent does not mean "gone forever" (that is, the mother who leaves the room and can no longer be seen is still alive). According to modern viewpoints, this concept is acquired in the second or at the latest the third year of life, if not earlier. It certainly is not delayed until the age of six to eight, although that is what Piaget assumed when he originated the concept.

From an addition to a 1919 reprint of *The Interpretation of Dreams*, which was originally published in 1913, we can discern that the matter may not have been entirely unambiguous even for Freud. He told of a four-year-old child who wishes that a servant girl who had annoyed him were dead. When his father asks if it wouldn't suffice if she simply left, the child answered that she might then come back again. At this point Freud understood that four-year-olds can already perceive a difference among the various forms of "absence."

Of course, Freud was not fundamentally opposed to a discussion about death. He was entirely in agreement that adults have to deal with death, and he expressed this clearly, probably in part due to the influence of World War I. In 1915 in his *Reflections on War and Death,* he closed with the following words:

> Shall we not admit that in our civilized attitude towards death we have again lived psychologically beyond our means? Shall we not turn around and avow the truth? Were it not better to give death the place to which it is entitled both in reality and in our thoughts and to reveal a little more of our unconscious attitude towards death which up to now we have so carefully suppressed? This may not appear a very high achievement and in some respects rather a step backwards, a kind of regression, but at least it has the advantage of taking the truth into account a little more and of making life more bearable again. To bear life remains, after all, the first duty of the living. The illusion becomes worthless if it disturbs us in this. We remember the old saying, "Si vis pacem, para bellum"—"If you wish peace, prepare for war." The times call for a paraphrase, "Si vis vitam, para mortem"—"If you wish life, prepare for death."

With this formulation, Freud was certainly a trailblazer for the idea of confronting and dealing with death, an idea that is still controversial to this day. In 1973, Ernst Becker wrote in his book *The Denial of Death,* "Man is literally split in two: he has an awareness of his own splendid uniqueness in that he sticks out of nature with a towering majesty, and yet he goes back into the ground a few feet in order blindly and dumbly to rot and disappear forever. It is a terrifying dilemma to be in and to have to live with."

From Freud's perspective, this is not a reason to go insane. And Martin Heidegger (quoted in Elschenbroich 2002) was more or less of Freud's opinion when he stated that death and absolute nothingness are constantly before man's inner eye and that life only acquires its true meaning through the omnipresent knowledge of inevitable death. Of course, for whatever reason, he never wrote anything about children.

I discuss these controversial ideas at length here to remind us that both adults and children confront their own deaths only occasionally and often only to a limited extent. Freud remarked that nobody can think constantly about his own death. But in the final analysis there is no fundamental difference between adults and children in this regard. Dealing with death and developing concepts of death begin very early in life, and both Freud and Jean Piaget were wrong when they fundamentally denied children these two capabilities.

Jean Piaget studied the cognitive and intellectual development of children intensively in the 1920s (Cousinet 1939; Cotton and Range 1990). He used the term *animism* to describe the mental phenomenon in children that causes them to ascribe lifelike qualities to inanimate objects (Piaget 1978). His use of this term contrasts with that of earlier anthropologists, who used it to mean the distinction between subject and object, between body and soul. In Piaget's case, animism was created not through the separation of object and subject but through a fusion of the two; the child is connected to the stone to which it ascribes life. In practice, the underlying cause is a defective border between the child and his environment. The concept implies that the object is an extension of the subject. Using this model, according to Piaget, we can see the development of animism in children take place in four stages. The sequence of these stages is fixed, but the age at which a child reaches the next stage can vary depending on individual and cultural differences or experiences.

At first, everything is alive that is active in any way. In the next phase, it is movement that causes something to seem alive. Since cars move, they are alive. The next step is characterized by active or spontaneous movement. A car needs a driver and therefore isn't alive. And in the last phase of this development, the child recognizes that only plants and animals are alive. According to Piaget, the first stage lasts into the sixth or seventh year for the majority of Swiss children, and the second stage occurs between six and eight. Between the ages of eight and eleven, children recognize that life is limited to plants and animals.

I. Huang and H. W. Lee (1945) rejected the idea of a type of logic specific to children that leads to various types of animism. For these authors, a child is different from an adult only because he or she lacks certain information about the real world. A stone seems alive to children only because they haven't been taught anything else. A. Strauss contradicted this view some years later after he had studied the authors' ideas and supported Piaget's view instead. Strauss posited a construct of four stages in the development of children's thought that can be summarized as follows (according to Deutsch 1937):

- in the first year: sensorimotor development to the point of anticipating the results of actions
- from one to two years: preoperational, graphical thinking
- from five to six years: concrete-operational thinking
- about twelve years and up: formal-operational thinking

For Piaget, this development was the result of an individual's continuous confrontation with the environment. Its steps, as he saw them, are climbed in a certain order. Reaching a lower step is the prerequisite for climbing to the next one. In the first stage, the child lacks any possibility of reflecting on nonbeing. In Piaget's view, the concept of object permanence, acquired between the sixth and eighth months of life, is actually an obstacle to developing an idea of death in the second phase, preoperational thinking. The child knows that his mother, whom he can't see any more, is still alive. The logical consequence would be that in the ideas of children, even dead people are still living and are just away temporarily.

In the final stage of sensorimotor development, children are already able to anticipate the results of their actions, and acting is of central importance at this age. The idea of causal processes without an actor, however, still presents difficulties. So natural events or diseases are candidates as causes of death in a child's mind, because they (diseases, for example) are active. In contrast, children cannot understand death as the natural end of an aging process, but they do understand it as the result of an action, of killing. But since an understanding of the difference between living and dead is still absent, children cannot imagine the final end of all life functions or the universality of death.

Consequently, in the stage of concrete-operational thinking it becomes possible for children to differentiate among the living, the dead, and the inanimate. They can differentiate between dying and being killed. But the ideas of the universality of death and of death as a result of the termination of all life processes is still alien to children at this stage, and the idea that they themselves can die has not yet entered their consciousness.

In the final stage—roughly after the age of twelve—children's thinking gets closer and closer to an adult's world of imagination, according to Strauss (as well as Piaget). The timing of the transition from concrete-operational to formal-operational thinking is probably variable, since Piaget does not cite a precise age, as he did for the early stages.

Concepts of death, as I stated before, cannot be separated from concepts of life. Piaget cited more precise ages for the development of ideas about life than for those about death (Cousinet 1939; Bowlby 1980). From the third to the sixth year of life, everything is alive that possesses activity or function. This is the principle of active acting, which is inherent even in fire, for example. From the sixth to the eighth year of life, everything is alive that moves, and the border between biology and mechanics still seems to be difficult. From the eighth to the twelfth year of life, everything is designated alive that supplies its own motion, and after the twelfth year only plants, animals, and people are considered alive.

His theory of developmental stages shows us why Piaget thought children could not produce a realistic concept of death until approximately age twelve. These ideas strongly influenced developmental psychologists and doctors in subsequent decades. Many later studies of the development of children's death concepts are based on this multistage model, and their hypotheses are based on levels of cognitive development. The assumption that children don't enter the realm of adult ideas at all until they are twelve definitely helped medicine cling for so long to the belief that children do not think about death. And so it was never necessary to talk with sick children about the fact that (sooner or later) they will have to die.

In 1934, Paul Schilder and David Wechsler published a study of seventy-six children aged five to fifteen, some healthy, some mentally ill. The study employed the "question-discussion method" supplemented by a special type of play and an image test. They used questions that had been developed for testing adults in the framework of a structured interview. Giving an answer didn't involve the subject's belief or opinion but rather his inner perceptions (introspection). For studying children, particularly younger ones, this is not workable. The content of the question must be discussed with the children in order to find out what experience they have had.

Schilder and Wechsler mentioned, for example, that we can't simply ask what ideas or mental images the children have when they think about death. Instead, you have to ask them, "What happens when a person dies?" or "Would you like to die?" or "Is dying painful?" They came to the conclusion that children's notions about death consist primarily of the idea of deprivation. Death isn't the natural end of life; it is seen instead as an event that happens due to a violent act, particularly an act of mutilation. Children find it difficult to reconcile conventional and religious views of death with their own experiences, and they only succeed when they adopt the adults' views totally and uncritically. But children are realists, and they turn the conventional views they learn from adults into something concrete. Children live continuously in a world of verbal insecurities and mysterious insinuations full of threats and dangers. For children, the meaning of words is much more complex than the definitions we find in a dictionary. Many words that children hear for the first time are fragments of orders, rules, admonitions, or warnings from adults. General words like these don't define straightforward situations, nor do they remind us of objects; instead, they remind us of the experiences linked to them. Children try to evade these uncertainties and escape into concrete experiences. For them, a clearly defined experience from which they can generalize is enough to enable them to develop a realistic concept. The full meaning of words is often not clear to children, but they do understand the emotional content.

Children know from their own experience that people die, and they usually accept it. Of course they do not believe in their own death. Instead they see death as an event that happens to other people, who suffer a loss because of it (for example, the loss of a possession or of the affection of other people). The idea of their own death occurs at most in connection with violence that can cause people to die. Children's own aggressiveness, with which they live every day, makes violence comprehensible to them. For children, loss is usually not something permanent, so death too seems reversible to them.

In contrast to Piaget, Schilder and Wechsler dispensed with the multistage model, and they granted children a much greater ability to think independently. Their most important contribution, however, was to acknowledge the important role played by children's experience.

In 1939, the French psychologist Roger Cousinet published a study on children's ideas about death. First, he noted that up to that point it had, in effect, been only philosophers and novelists who had investigated people's ideas about death. For them, the word *death* is tied to a human emotional reaction and has no meaning in and of itself. Death means the end of life or represents the suffering that is triggered for us by someone's death. But for people who are not part of a philosophical (and religious?) or literary tradition or are not accustomed to psychological questions, the word *death* has no content, in Cousinet's view. He quoted Michel de Montaigne, who said, "Neither death nor life concerns you; life, because you exist, death because you no longer do." For such people, the thought of death means seeing themselves in someone else's death or dealing with their own distress, grief at being abandoned, or the balance sheet of someone else's life or of their own. This kind of thinking, according to Cousinet, is so universal that it also rubs off on children.

From this point of view, contact with death or with a dead or dying person is seen as an event that touches children's sensitivity. It is generally assumed that the blow is stronger for children than for adults, because everyone agrees that children are more fragile and sensitive. Cousinet's opinion is that nothing could be further from the truth. Children's sensitivity does not have the effect of stopping their intellectual activity; it has exactly the opposite effect. And for children, a new stimulus for intellectual activity is an impetus for a new mental construction. In all their speculations up to now, according to Cousinet, psychologists and psychoanalysts wanted us to believe that children lead a life without coherence caused by their deep ignorance and the weakness of their ability to think logically. He believed that children are far removed from being disturbed by emotions that arise from the depths of their own selves. Children constantly control and repress these emotions, prompted by all kinds of events and feelings they have experienced, without being compelled by some external authority. Organizing their mental life, their thinking and feeling, is a task of supreme importance for children; its goal is to create an orderly internal world, what Piaget characterized as "children's philosophical system."

Further, Cousinet added, it is a serious problem that children don't usually receive equivalent information about the phenomenon of death and the phenomenon of life. If a five-year-old asks how people come into the world, he often receives a clear answer. But if the same child wants to know how the living leave this world, he usually receives evasive answers.

Only the answer to the first question is in a seven-year-old's knowledge inventory today, as I pointed out earlier (Elschenbroich 2002). So following Cousinet's lead, we might ask, "What else can children do but construct their own explanatory system?" Up to this point, children's thinking has been nurtured and shaped only by experiences and perceptions that they have processed intellectually; now death penetrates this thinking. And this is a new and contradictory element, since it is not an object of experience or perception. This fact triggers an intellectual state of shock that unsettles their thinking in its entirety. Their first natural impulse is to reject this new element and keep it from entering the mind.

Cousinet then described how ideas about death develop in several stages, using a six-year-old as an example. According to the child's first notion, death is like a bad illness, worse than all the others, but which can be cured under certain circumstances. Admittedly, these circumstances are not easy to come by. The second idea, in which death occurs in two stages, comes closer to reality. First a "preliminary" death occurs, a condition that may last months or years, during which the child is cared for. Only then does definitive death arrive. This way, the child approaches the truth and moves naturally from myth to reality. Finally, in the third stage, the child develops a realistic image of death. Nonbeing finds a place in the child's mental world, and death is no longer, as it was in the first stage of understanding, a simple negation. In this stage, the child's thinking functions unhindered, and death acquires a positive value. If the child has finally accepted death's existence, then he or she takes an intensive look at it and poses questions. The age at which that happens differs greatly from one child to another, according to Cousinet. He doesn't specify ages but assumes an earlier age than did Piaget—before age twelve in any case.

Cousinet, it should be mentioned, did not study a large number of children; in his 1939 article, he used the example of one six-year-old as evidence for his statements. He came to two conclusions:

- The evolution of the idea of death in children's thinking progresses from abstract to concrete. First, it is an abstraction, detached from any actual context. Death is like a cessation or a separation. Incrementally, this abstraction becomes unthinkable, and step by step the concept is filled out with concrete elements.
- In the case of children, the essential fact is that they continuously intensify their lives, and they want to continue to live this life, which is a necessary foundation and the reason for being. Now death becomes one element of life. Through a reversal, through a reconstruction that means a tremendous exertion for their thinking, the children transform the negation into being. This transformation occurs through a quasi-scientific effort of analysis. The brutal, incomprehensible fact disintegrates into a certain number of concrete elements. Each of these elements is the object of an investigation through questions that are sufficient to satisfy intellectual curiosity or through imitative action in play that permits a more complete assimilation. Credit for all this work is due to the remarkable life force of children, not to their intelligence. This capability is one of the essential elements in children's thinking.

Why go into Cousinet's work in such detail? It is fascinating because at an early date, taking Piaget's ideas into account, it describes the development of a concept of death as a continuous process within children's thinking. But Cousinet did not agree with Piaget that the developmental stages are rigid, with minimal possibilities for deviation. He made it clear how individual this development is as well as the role played by impressions and experience. He consciously avoided giving ages. And his work makes one more extremely important point: he acknowledged that children have the intellectual capacity to develop concepts of life and death at a very early age. Children are not at all disturbed when a new factor enters their thought process. Cousinet's work is a call to respect children's thinking and emotions and not to persist with the old notion that children lead "a life characterized by disjointedness." Understanding this is a precondition if we want to support children who are seriously ill or dying. In comparison with Piaget, Cousinet's 1939 article pointed in the direction of doing greater justice to children.

A multistage model like that of Piaget was posited by A. Gesell and L. Ilg in 1946 (Carey 1985). While Piaget based his concept on the development of thinking, these authors focused on how emotional response develops. Their greatly expanded series of stages has to be viewed somewhat skeptically, since its empirical basis is not optimal, but their findings provide an addition to Piaget's concepts. They too pointed out that care should be exercised in using a strict age scale.

For the authors we have reviewed up to this point, studying children's development of a concept of death was only a component of their broader research on child development in general. In 1949 the English psychologist Sylvia Anthony published a book that dealt specifically with the awareness of death in childhood. It was the result of a three-year study using projective tests on a small, carefully controlled group of children. Many lines of thought and deliberations were adopted from studies by earlier researchers, but additional aspects were also investigated. Anthony was convinced that the maturation of a concept of death depends on the level of intellectual development, not on chronological age. The young child thinks about death as a form of aggression or separation or as a combination of the two. The result is the development of anxieties in every case, so it would be a mistake to assume that young children are free of anxiety. Anthony also noted that some children under age seven make accepting their own death easier through an active process

of denial—a phenomenon familiar to us in the world of adults but here described with regard to relatively young children.

In 1943 A. Weber published an article about work done in a pediatric psychiatric observation ward in a Swiss canton. He shared the widely held opinion that the experience of death plays little or no role for children who grew
up, as these did, in happy and peaceful circumstances. He justified the conventional wisdom as follows, that

> one's own death is further away from childhood than from other ages, and a
> happy child growing up under the protection of his parents has no reason to
> worry much more about it. Children's thinking is generally incapable of grasp-
> ing the meaning and seriousness of death, possibly not until puberty. . . . Things
> change with puberty. With sexual maturity, death accompanies love into the
> realm of experience as its antithesis and dark background. Like the longed-for
> final self-surrender in love, death is viewed as the deliverer, releasing us from
> the self, grown problematic for the first time, and acting as guide to a mysteri-
> ous new being. Death is often linked to love or even mistaken for it in the world
> of imagination, may even follow after it in deeds. For the person beset by world-
> weariness and existential anxiety, death seems to be the final safe refuge.

Weber noted that up to that point, little attention had been paid to how
children relate to death. He pursued interesting questions in his investigation. He included three case reports plus the results of a survey of sixty mildly
to severely neurotic hospitalized children; he supplemented these data with
his experiences with the other children in the same ward and with fifteen
hundred primary school children in Bern examined as outpatients. That
these children are ill, he emphasized, does not diminish the value of the evidence; on the contrary, some things stand out even more clearly.

The children ranged in age from 4 years, 9 months to 15 years, 1 month.
Without exception, they expressed fear of dying. Few of them were able to
give clear reasons for their fear, although some tried to do so using stories
they had heard from adults. But the naturalness and directness of what they
said convinced Weber that they couldn't possibly have borrowed or learned it
from adults. As they expressed it, it was fear of a transformation into a new,
uncertain, strange, in any case unpleasant condition that was inferior to
their vigorous, active life. It was all the things you couldn't do if you were
dead that mainly determined their aversion, and it was not much comfort
that dying didn't hurt, as many believed. Weber reported that very few men-

tioned separation from their families, who would then cry. When he spoke with the children about their own death, the younger ones weren't thinking about the rest of the world at all; their own well-being absorbed all their attention. They felt a lot of sympathy with other children who were dying.

Weber learned that the children's answers often provided good information about their background, education, surroundings, and personality or about their attitude toward family members. This illustrates again how problematic it is to generalize too much. The children portrayed death as a strange, eerie condition in which darkness surrounds you and you can no longer do anything. Weber emphasizes that their ideas don't differ from those of adults in clarity or lack thereof. Death and sleep were described as similar by almost all of the children.

Weber observed that a probing examination of death occurs in children of kindergarten age and later, during puberty, but remains dormant in the years between. Preoccupation with death proceeds much like preoccupation with questions of sexuality. Toddlers are inevitably confronted with death and dying in nature as they begin to walk and talk; it isn't surprising that their fear forces an intense confrontation with this vital question, as with others. According to Weber's observations, even toddlers can mourn for months; it is often overlooked because no one thinks they are capable of it. As Weber summarized his experiences with the fifteen hundred school children, there is no doubt that children experience the death of someone important to them with feelings that are autonomous, deep, and sustained, just as adults do.

The observations and surveys that Weber described are similar in many respects to Piaget's ideas. They do make clear, however, that the developmental stages defined by Piaget cannot be linked so clearly to specific ages and that children generally know more than people think. The point here is not to deny the value of Piaget's work in any fundamental way. I discuss the rigid series of steps posited by Piaget so extensively here because his successors have often taken the developmental stages he described too literally—and still do to this day. For a long time, this view has reinforced the fundamental opinion that children don't begin to develop realistic concepts of death until they are approximately twelve years old, an opinion that has not been especially helpful to children who are ill.

In 1948, the Hungarian psychologist Maria Nagy published a classic study in which she considered how children aged three to ten think about death.

She studied 378 healthy children using essays, drawings, and conversations. She identified three age-based developmental stages:

- 3–5 years: Children do not recognize that death is regular and final. Death means parting but also living on under different conditions. They imagine that death is only temporary or that there are different stages of death. Children know that they are living beings, but they do not yet distinguish between "alive" and "lifeless."
- 5–9 years: Death is now personified. Death occurs only occasionally and is not yet universal. If death exists for children, it is a person they try to keep at a distance: it is "Death," the one who "does it." And they have no answer for the question of why he "does it," if it's so bad for people. Death only carries away the people who die. Some children imagine that death and the dead person are identical, so they logically use the word *death* for dead people. The egocentric and anthropocentric thinking characteristic of the first years of life continues to play a role.
- After age 9: children recognize that death is a process that happens within us and accompanies the end of physical life. At this age, children know that death is unavoidable. Their concept of death is just as realistic as their general conception of the world.

Many elements of Nagy's statements are in accordance with Piaget's theory. In contrast to him, however, the age scale is clearly lowered from twelve to nine years with respect to a definite concept of death. It becomes clear once again how changeable children's views are and how problematic an inflexible age scale is in this area. There are of course twenty years separating the publications of the two authors. Nagy emphasized at the end of her article that it is impossible to hide death from children and that we should not try to do so. Behaving naturally when we interact with children, she felt, can greatly help to minimize the shock caused when they do encounter death. This early study confirms that as adults we need to allow children the opportunity to deal with death at an early age and that we are not doing them any favors by preventing it.

In 1957 the German child psychiatrist Erich Stern published the valuable book he had written during his exile in France under the title *Kind, Krankheit und Tod* (The child, illness, and death). His ideas about children's knowledge are rooted deeply in Piaget's teachings. Nevertheless, he engaged in his own intensive search for specific indications of how children understand death. He reported on children who saw death during air raids, for example, or who had lost one or both of their parents. Children as young as four clearly showed that they were afraid of death. Fear of death was obviously especially pronounced in Jewish children who were hiding in France and feared constantly for their lives. Many of these children lived with substantial anxieties that required therapy. He closed the chapter with the following notable conclusions: "Taken together, these cases are very interesting and above all extremely remarkable from a clinical perspective; they require a lengthy and intensive involvement with the child, a psychotherapy with the goal of resolving anxiety. We considered only recent observations; there would certainly be more cases in our medical data. But as important and interesting as they may be, these are isolated observations, and they provide very little specific information about the development of children's ideas about death. Isolated observations appear to be insufficient."

Stern reported extensively about studies of healthy children and encountered developmental concepts that we know from other authors such as Freud and Piaget. He concluded that children in general do not think about death. This doesn't change until they enter adolescence; in principle, young people know about death at that point. But adolescents don't relate the eventuality of death to themselves. Stern asserted that this is true even when a fellow patient dies whom the adolescent knows well. He reported, however, that he practiced for some time in a sanatorium where he got to know dying adolescents from a working-class background. He had intensive conversations about dying with these young people and noticed with admiration that they had a much more natural attitude toward death than the "intellectuals," for example. In his opinion, this is also true for adults. Stern ascribed the young people's attitude to their Catholic background, since Catholics believe that our own death has a meaning for the salvation of others. In Stern's view, this is a naive belief that helps people accept death.

Stern reported at length about the young people's different behavior patterns when confronted with death. Some remain indifferent; death is no concern of theirs. For them, death lies in the distant future. Some react with a more or less brutal cynicism, which is intended to hide their own fear. For another type of adolescent, a mood dominated by world-weariness produces a longing for death, which is usually overcome quickly. For young people whose emotions are unstable, however, this can lead to serious consequences, such as suicide. Stern, an experienced psychiatrist, reported about his conversations with adolescents, yet he did not encourage his readers to talk about death with people who are dying. He believed that the majority of young people, including Catholics from a higher social stratum, don't want to hear about death; adolescents with a Catholic working-class background are the exception.

Irving Alexander and Arthur Adlerstein (1958) used an approach that was both interesting and completely different from the researchers we have discussed up to this point. They wanted to find out how children of different ages react emotionally to the idea of death. They studied 108 boys between the ages of five and sixteen. Their method used a word association exercise; they recorded the response time, the galvanic skin response, and the answer itself. Variations in the answers in response to "basal" words (for example, *dress, brave, happy, star, speech, animal*) and words with the stem "death" (*death, dead, deathlike*) were intended to provide information about emotional associations with regard to death. Children in all three age groups (5–8, 9–12, 13–16) reacted to death-related words with increased latency and diminished skin resistance in comparison to the basal words.

Alexander and Adlerstein found substantial variation with regard to age. The latency time probably reflects the cultural situation, while the changes in skin resistance are more likely a reflection of inner feelings. It is interesting to note that there was an age-dependent increase in both these parameters for the entire group, but no change for skin resistance in the middle group. According to the authors, children in this age group have a stable ego and are so busy with normal everyday life that they can't think about death. This would explain why they have so little emotional response. Alexander and Adlerstein interpreted their data as follows: There is nothing special about childhood in comparison to later life that triggers an elevated emotional response to death. Instead, the ego's stability decreases due to increased psychological stress in the youngest and oldest age groups, in contrast to the 9–12 group. The result is a heightened emotional reaction to death in these groups.

Gwen Safier (1964) studied the connection between Nagy's stages in the development of a death concept and Piaget's theory of animism. She found an unambiguous correlation between the concepts of life and death, which run parallel in their development. The older children become, the less they tend to connect life or death with an object. A certain fuzziness is typical of the group of children aged seven to eight (admittedly, there were only ten children in each group). The author explained this with Piaget's view that seven-year-old children are in a transitional phase during which they shift from a global to an analytical approach to thinking. These findings confirm Alexander and Adlerstein's observations (1958), although they saw the explanation in the strong ego typical for this age group.

Children's Grief

To approach the development of children's concept of death from another perspective, we can ask whether children are able to grieve and, if they can, at what age this becomes possible. Because grieving is closely tied to the ability to develop a concept of death, a brief discussion of children's grieving process is appropriate here; the literature cited in the bibliography provides a more extensive discussion of this topic.

A. Hahn (1968) defined grief as the subjective reaction to the loss of something felt to be irreplaceable. Death, which he described as a total, irreparable truncation of all current reciprocal connections with another person, is just such an event. The word *mourning* is used in psychoanalysis to describe the psychological process set in motion by the loss of a beloved object. John Bowlby (1960b) discussed this topic in one of his studies. He referred to Donald Winnicott (1954), who wanted to use this expression only for cases that are part of a positive development. He was opposed—correctly, I think—when researchers within an academic discipline impose multiple meanings on a single term. So in what follows, I use Bowlby's definition, which addresses a broad spectrum of psychological processes triggered by loss.

Early on, psychoanalysts held the opinion that weaning and the loss of the mother's breast was not only the first loss a child experienced but also the most significant, from the viewpoint of pathology. Since children are usually weaned during the first year, everyone concluded that the decisive phase during which children develop the ability to work through a loss successfully also occurred during the first months of life (Klein 1936). Bowlby believed that Melanie Klein and others had attached too much importance to weaning and that traumas such as the loss of affection or even the loss of the mother have a much more far-reaching effect. Of course children experience weaning as a loss, but it is not the decisive experience. The period during which weaning occurs extends for quite some time. It begins at approximately six months and lasts into the fourth year or even longer. Bowlby is convinced that children can experience separation anxiety and grief during this entire period that can substantially change the development of their personalities.

Bowlby elaborated on this complex of problems at length and gave examples of how young children work through separation from (loss of) their mother (Robertson and Bowlby 1952; Bowlby 1958, 1960a, 1980). An initial period during which they may protest and demand that their mother return may last for many days, but then children calm down. One gets the impression they have forgotten their parents. I can remember very well that this opinion was widely held in children's hospitals during the 1960s and 1970s. Working together with the British group around Bowlby, French authors reached the same conclusions with respect to children between twelve and seventeen months. They showed the same behavior patterns in children and confirmed that these sometimes have effects that extend over long periods of time (Roudinesco et al. 1952). The hostility that develops with a persistent longing for the mother is often ignored, although it was described in the early 1950s by Heinicke (1956).

Loss of the mother occasioned by a stay in the hospital is a traumatic experience for young children. It is not realistic to expect them to be happy about the care they are receiving from the doctors and hospital staff and not to grieve about the loss of their mother (Bowlby et al. 1952; Robertson and Bowlby 1952). It was difficult to admit this at the time and develop approaches that were appropriate. Today we can hardly imagine the practice common in those days of not allowing parents to visit their children in the hospital.

John Robertson (1953) reported on many cases of young children whose longing for their mothers was evident over a long period of time. He also pointed out that this persistent reaction can easily be overlooked. Anna Freud and Dorothy Burlingham (1943) also described many toddlers who displayed clear signs of grief. They claimed that this reaction is short-lived, particularly in children under two, and thus differs clearly from adult grief. Anna Freud contradicted Bowlby's claim that children even as young as six months can grieve (Freud 1969). In fact, Bowlby's and Robertson's observations prove something else. Young children too can obviously grieve for a long time. Helene Deutsch (1937) expressed the opinion early on that children, in contrast to adults, are not able to complete the grieving process. It was her hypothesis that a child's ego is not sufficiently developed to withstand the strain of grieving. So children use the mechanism of narcissistic self-protection to avoid the grieving process. In an article published in 1953, Rochlin too denied that children are actually capable of grieving. He did not claim, however, that children are not stressed by a loss. But in his opinion, they don't react with depression or arrogance, as adults do; instead they display other clinical phenomena or developmental disorders.

Bowlby discussed the various findings in the psychoanalytic literature, pointing finally to two fundamental and contentious issues. The first is the fundamental question of whether children do or do not consciously experience a loss, and if they do, at what point they go through a phase of grieving. The second follows if we accept that there is such a reaction, namely what must the nature of the beloved object be in order for it to trigger grief. He summarized as follows: Grief and its sustained psychological process are present in very young children and are linked closely with separation anxiety. And it is the loss of the mother, not the loss of the breast during weaning, that is the more important event in the life of a young child.

At the beginning of this section I mentioned that the ability to grieve is closely tied to the presence of a concept of death. Robert Furman's experience shows that children who were not able to deal with death emotionally at first contact were able to do so at second contact after a short time had passed (Furman 1965). It appears that children use the first experience to develop a concept of death. It is true that some two-year-olds already have such a concept, while many five-year-olds do not. Furman thought that this fact explained many of the differences in the literature. Grieving is no different. Many children are clearly in a position to grieve at an early age, while others are not as far along in their development or experience. He believed, however, that we can expect children's ego function to be mature enough between the ages of two and three for them to understand the meaning of death. He also believed that other maturation processes must be added to the ability to conceptualize death for an effective grieving process to be possible.

So how should we respond to children's grief? I do not doubt that children, even very young children, are able to grieve. I remember a three-year-old girl, whose cancer was no longer treatable, who painted pictures of graves over and over again. She had often been at the cemetery with her mother to visit her grandmother's grave. When we asked the child what these pictures were supposed to represent, she answered that she didn't know, she was just very sad. And that was exactly what she communicated to the team in the weeks preceding her death. It was evident that not only was she able to grieve, she was even capable of anticipatory grief as well. She was able to grieve over her own approaching death. The less we keep knowledge about their own death from children, the more intensively they will be prompted to this kind of anticipatory grieving process, which will enable them to accept the death-related loss of self and of objects (Solnit 1965).

According to Janis (quoted in Bürgin 1978), an anticipatory anxiety starts as soon as the threat is perceived. This anxiety may have a positive effect, because it leads to a mobilization of psychological resources, causes a heightening of discriminatory vigilance, and encourages the need to seek and accept help. A preparatory grieving process is linked to this psychological work (Bürgin 1978). And children are already capable of this. We should not deny children the ability to grieve, as we often do, for example, when we don't allow them to participate in funerals because we think that they, in contrast to adults, don't have any need for a mourning ritual.

In his remarkable article "On the Dying of Death," Robert Fulton (1967) wrote that wise management of grief concentrates on two central things in the case of both children and adults: encouraging and easing the normal grieving process and averting a delayed or false grieving process. He also emphasized that the funeral ritual eases the work of grieving if it conforms to the social and psychological requirements of the survivors. Participating enables a child to understand that death has occurred and that he or she is one among many people who are suffering because of it. And the child may also experience consolation and affection from family members that they would otherwise have missed. Children are sometimes afraid that they were involved in causing the death; others can help them recognize their own innocence. If children are experiencing a crisis because of the death, being excluded from the funeral can reinforce the idea that they must have done something wrong. When the funeral is over, children often continue to be excluded from the community of mourners. For this reason, Fulton emphasized in closing the importance of making it possible for children to work through their grief.

Denial leads to a pathological grieving process. Fathers of deceased children in particular tend to continue functioning "normally" at any cost, leaving no room for grieving. I can remember the father of a child who died of leukemia; he continued to meet his professional responsibilities without interruption, but privately he spoke less and less, until after six months he fell completely silent. Soon thereafter he attempted suicide, claiming that he too was sick with leukemia and had to join his daughter. This kind of pathological grieving process also occurs with children; of course the result makes less of an impression on the outside world, with the result that it can easily be overlooked.

After having thoroughly considered the possibilities children have for grieving, we need to return to the topic of children's concepts of death. In 1965, Furman was already suggesting that children are able to deal with death at a very early age. At the same time, he emphasized the variability among personalities and the important influence of personal experience. He asked at what age we should help children understand death, and how we can do so. He believed that a two- or three-year-old child is very much in a position to understand the possibility of his or her own death if, for example, his or her mother talks honestly about the loss of objects that are familiar to the child. Many parents fulfill this task only if circumstances force them to, in times of war, for example (Freud and Burlingham 1943). Usually parents postpone it until the child has to cope with a real loss, such as the death of a grandmother. We have to realize that this forces children to fulfill two tasks at the same time—coming to terms with death and working through the loss of their grandmother—and many children are successful in doing so. Fulton suggested in this context that parents should seek professional help from psychologists, psychiatrists, or pediatricians with pertinent experience when the loss is a serious one that affects them too, such as the suicide of one of the child's parents, for example. Usually the other parent is so overwhelmed that he or she can be of help only in a limited way, if at all.

In 1966, Marjorie Editha Mitchell published her book *The Child's Attitude to Death*, in which she provided an outstanding critical summary of the current state of knowledge about children's attitude to death. She had learned that immobility is the most important aspect of death for children, confirming the observations of earlier authors (Illig and Bates-Ames 1955). She wrote extensively about the connection between sleep and death, something that had concerned the Roman poet Virgil, who had characterized sleep as the brother of death. Death cements the feared link among sleep, separation, darkness, and death. Mitchell explained that sleep is the end of each day's life. I return to this point later during the discussion of children's frequent question about what it's like to die. The answer I often gave as a young doctor, that dying is exactly like falling asleep, acquires an unpleasant aftertaste when considered in this context. After I realized this and observed children who became afraid of going to sleep as a result, I never again used these "comforting words."

Mitchell confirmed the developmental stages posited by Piaget, but she also questioned the accuracy of his age scale. She believed that five-year-olds already link the disappearance and disintegration of the body with death. For children who grow up on a farm, this happens even earlier. Here we see the importance of experience, something that was not sufficiently observed or considered by either psychoanalysis or Piaget. Mitchell was also convinced that children are interested in learning something about death even before they are six. She emphasized that we have to consider what strong disagreements there are in our society about the connection between death and all sorts of fear and hope. In this context, it is extremely difficult to find out how children's ideas develop. When fear of death seems to be intensive and immature, many psychologists tend to view it as psychopathic. It is a sign of self-preoccupation if it persists into adulthood. Mitchell wondered how we can hope to find out anything at all about how children think in a society in which no one talks about death with children.

In 1967, a study by Wayne Gartley and Marion Bernasconi confirmed earlier findings by Paul Schilder and David Wechsler (1934) to the effect that children are able to deal with death in a realistic way. But they found no evidence to confirm that children between five and nine imagine a physical embodiment of death (Nagy 1948). They concluded that children accept death as a fact—better as they get older—and that they acquire a fear of death only by observing adults. Gartley and Bernasconi were also not able to confirm that young children saw death as being reversible. According to their interpretation, an early religious education as well as television accustomed children earlier to the realities of death than had been the case in the past. They concluded, "It appears to be true that a simple and open explanation is more advisable than an attempt to conceal death from children."

Explaining Death to Children, edited by Earl A. Grollmann (1967), was unusual for its time. Louise Bates Ames (1958) wrote these opening words to the book, "If you know exactly what you'd say to a child of any age faced for the first time by the death of someone very close to him, and if you yourself have a clear and comfortable understanding of death and what it means, you don't need a book on the subject." This is a remarkable statement, if only because so little has changed since then. We all have to admit that we are still struggling with the same issues, although we have learned a lot in the last forty years. The book's ten chapters expose a broad spectrum of topics, and it is notable that three of the chapters were written by Protestant, Catholic, and

Jewish clergy (Grollman 1967a; Jackson 1967; Riley 1967). It would be interesting to illuminate the subject of this book against a religious backdrop, but that would be outside its scope. Therefore I discuss briefly only three other chapters from the book by Grollmann.

The first chapter, by Robert Fulton, deals with death in a broad sense. He emphasized that in 1960s America, death was no longer viewed as the unavoidable result of original sin; instead, it is an avoidable and unnecessary misfortune, the result of personal negligence and unanticipated accidents. He gave his article the interesting title "On the Dying of Death." This topic is treated generally and not as it relates to children, so a detailed discussion is not appropriate here; his insistence on the necessity of mourning work for children was discussed earlier.

In the second chapter, Gregory Rochlin discussed how young children perceive themselves and death. In earlier articles (1953, 1959), Rochlin had reported that the fear of losing important people such as parents and the fear of being abandoned are clearly identifiable even in young children. Adults and children like to avoid the topic of death, and from this Rochlin concluded that adults are not a good source of information for children. Nevertheless, even young children already know about death. Under normal circumstances, they make discoveries about death early on and have ample additional opportunities to acquire information.

Rochlin thought that there is no doubt that young children learn quickly that death is the absence of life, and that with it, life ends. And the better children understand this, the more uncertain they become about the future. They have already experienced frustration and not having their wishes fulfilled and have learned how to deal with that. Although they recognize the reality of death, young children do not yet show any pragmatic or philosophical acceptance. But children have developed and perfected defense mechanisms when earlier conflicts arose, and these make it possible for them to deal with difficult situations. This involves two psychological processes. The first enables them to modify an unpleasant awareness of something—of death, for example. The second process brings about a change in subjective experience in order to cope with helplessness and the sense of loss through fantasies of omnipotence and invulnerability. Many of these mechanisms have their source in a denial of reality. The disavowal and denial of the end of life in death is typical not just for children but for adults as well. Human beings clearly begin to confront death at a very early age, and at an equally early age they begin to deny it.

Rochlin was irritated that no studies of these fundamental issues had appeared in the two decades following Maria Nagy's work (1948). So he decided to demonstrate that death is an important topic with which even very young children are concerned. Other authors cited above had already pointed this out, but Rochlin wanted to show that this was not out of the ordinary. So he studied a group of healthy children, selected according to the following criteria: They had to be between three and five years old; they had to demonstrate, during a play session, organized thinking that was expressed both verbally and in play; and they had to be from urban families with well-educated parents who had no close ties to the church. He excluded children who grew up in the country because of their early exposure to birth, life, and death. All of the children were of average intelligence and had no exacerbating circumstances such as separation, serious illness, or other hardships within their immediate families.

The results can be summarized as follows. The studies confirmed Rochlin's view that children have defense mechanisms that enable them to confront death and dying without being put at risk. Magical thinking—the idea that we can bring about certain events through our thoughts, words, and actions—still plays a big role at this age. The children often overcome their fear of death as they do other fears, through repetitive play situations. The denial can be so complete that it leads to a complete negation of something that has happened. Children understand death as a shutdown of the vital functions. They view these functions as important for life in general and as essential for themselves. Moral factors appear early on: an evil person dies earlier than a good person, and good people are allowed to come back again. The serious meaning of death isn't hidden from the children. They know that in the end death is unavoidable, they seem to learn early that life ends at that point, and they apply this knowledge to themselves.

Rochlin wrote,

> To expect that the child would entertain adult conceptions of dying or death would not only be unreasonable but naïve. The facts of death like the facts of life, however, are to the child heavily embossed with every conscious and unconscious emotion at his disposal. These psychological vicissitudes do not serve the ends of reality, but rather quite opposite ends. The incentive to repress the real significance of dying may be judged from the powerful mental mechanisms which are brought into function in order to transcend death. What is remarkable is not that children arrive at adult views of the cessation of life, but rather

how tenaciously throughout life adults hold to the child's beliefs and how readily they revert to them. The clinical facts show that the child's views of dying
and death are inseparable from the psychological defenses against the reality of
death. They form a hard matrix of beliefs which is shaped early and deep in emotional life. It appears not to alter throughout life. The concept of death fused
with its amalgam of defenses is established as a core, around which a knowledge
of the facts of life is wrapped. The knowledge will vary considerably in people
and in different societies and cultures, but neither the core nor the defenses differ in any appreciable way. The core seems to be irreducible and unaltered.

The book's third chapter is titled "The Child's Understanding of Death:
How Does it Develop?" The author, Robert Kastenbaum, believed that many
young children go through a phase in which they talk about death openly, in
a matter-of-fact way and without any overlay of sorrow or anxiety. But these
very same children become adults who are speech-inhibited whenever the
topic of death is raised and who offer their own children only clichés and
evasions in explanation. This shows that children have to develop their concepts in a world that has not solved its own intellectual and emotional relationship with death. There are data available in the literature, Kastenbaum
assumed, that provide sufficient evidence that young children still lack most
of the mental operational mechanisms that would enable them to develop a
concept of their own death. Separation is the only exception. Even if we assume that children under the age of one do not yet have their own concept of
death, they still begin at a very early age to gather experiences and possibly
even experiment with an idea of death.

A. Maurer (1966) wrote that a child of three months is so comfortable in his
own sense of self that he begins to experiment with it. When a child hides
playfully behind a chair and then suddenly reappears, calling, "Peek-a-boo,"
he or she is in a secure situation, shifting between fear and pleasure. This and
other similar hiding games are not just games; they are also a formula for establishing yourself as an autonomous individual. Maurer interpreted young
children's interest in games that involve hiding and reappearing as little experiments with nonbeing or with death. He pointed to the interesting fact
that the English expression for this kind of game ("peek-a-boo") comes from
an Old English word that means "living or dead?" It is possible that toddlers
experiment with separation, loss, and nonbeing through play much more
than we realize, thus acquiring a basis for concepts they develop later.

Considering the findings in the literature, Maurer came to the following conclusions: thoughts about death are, in his opinion, closely tied from the very beginning to the total pattern of personality development, which itself is heavily influenced by the child's experience. It is artificial to conclude that development is completed in adolescence. It is instead a continuous process of maturation that lasts throughout life and does not conclude at some point in a full-blown concept. Although we reorganize our understanding of death repeatedly, we do not completely reject our earlier concepts; we go back to them again and again. As adults we can still view death through a child's eyes and personify it, for example.

In concluding this section about the book *Explaining Death to Children,* I quote Kastenbaum once more. He writes:

> We, as parents, have a superb opportunity to foster our children's development throughout their entire life-span—not simply for the next few years—by respecting their efforts to puzzle out the meaning of death. The more our children feel that they can approach us with their ideas on *any* subject and receive an interested, dependable hearing, then the more likely they are to share their meditations on death. A certain inner freedom and intellectual honesty is required on our own parts, is it not? Somehow we must keep developing and reevaluating our own orientations toward death if we are to be open and useful to our children in this area. We do not mean to leave the implication that parents should attempt to hurry their children through relatively early phases in the understanding of death. This advice has sometimes been given or implied by others. But we do not see any particular advantage in pressuring a youngster into being anything other than a natural person at his own age-level. If the subject of death does not embarrass or dismay us, if we can appreciate and respect the child's view of reality without losing our own, then we are in a position to foster his development through life with the beginnings of an enlightened orientation toward death.

By the middle of the 1960s, the idea that children develop concepts of death early on had become widespread in the literature of psychoanalysis. So Piaget's concept of stages could no longer be enlisted to argue that children are not able to deal with death, so no one can or must talk about death with them. As we will see, however, there was still no consensus about this issue at the beginning of the 1970s. In the next chapter, I describe the discussion of this topic that was beginning at the same time, albeit hesitantly, in the field of pediatrics. At this point, however, a discussion of the literature published during the past three decades in the fields of psychology and psychoanalysis is in order, since there have been new insights during this period.

In 1971, Perry Childers and Mary Wimmer reported on a study of seventy-three children between the ages of four and ten. They wanted to find out whether and at what point in time children understand the universality and the finality of death. How the children arrived at their knowledge played no role in the study. They concluded that children definitely do understand the universality of death and that this knowledge increases with age. In the youngest group (under six), only three of nineteen children were sure that death is a universal phenomenon; in the middle group (six to eight), nineteen of thirty-four children were; and in the oldest group (over nine), all the children were certain. There is no distinct age boundary, but after the age of eight or nine, all children are certain that death is universal. It is interesting to note that age-dependence for the idea of the finality of death was verifiable only to a limited extent; even some of the young children understood the meaning of finality. This study shows once again that we should avoid espousing a strict age scale with regard to concept development.

Humberto Nagera (1971) began his article by describing the controversial ideas in the research literature, pointing out that Wolf (1958) thought—much like Piaget—that concepts comparable to those of adults could not be identified in children before the age of ten or eleven. As I mentioned earlier, Furman (1960) clearly contradicted Wolf. At the same time, M. Wolfenstein (1966), using the ability to grieve as a starting point, had largely denied that children were able to develop a concept of death, and Nagera supported his findings. He summarized his own theories as follows: children experience only a short phase of sadness following a loss and are incapable of grieving for a longer period. He points to their distinct capacity for denial, their idea of death's reversibility, and their inability to understand the reality of death. Here he corroborated previous authors, discussed earlier in this book, who had denied that children could understand death.

Margot Tallmer and her collaborators (1974) investigated factors that influence children's concepts of death. They compared children from a low socio-economic class with children from the middle class and found that the former had a significantly more certain concept of death than the latter. In both groups, the development was clearly age-dependent. The authors speculated that children from a lower socioeconomic class are confronted with reality much earlier and more forcefully; television is also part of this reality, since the authors were convinced that television viewing among lower-class children is more frequent and less supervised. But in contrast to their preliminary assumptions, experience with violence does not play a big role. It is interesting to note that lower-class children develop both realistic concepts and the feelings that arise from them at an earlier age. This study demonstrates again that external factors play a role we should not disregard in children's development of concepts of death and thus reminds us once more to be careful about making generalizations.

In a study of children's concepts of death, Barbara Kane (1979) defined nine different components a concept can include:

- Realization of death
- Separation
- Immobility
- Finality
- Causality
- Dysfunctionality
- Universality
- Inability to feel
- Appearance of the dead person

She investigated which of these components are present and to what extent in children between three and twelve years of age. In her study of 122 healthy middle-class children, she came to six conclusions that can be summarized as follows:

- the components defined on the basis of the literature were confirmed by the study;
- understanding of the individual components developed in each case from being totally absent through being incompletely present to being completely present;
- concepts of death develop as a function of age;
- experience accelerates development only in children under six, not in older children;
- development occurs in three stages, analogous to Piaget's preoperational, concrete-operational and formal-operational stages; and
- all children over eight possess a concept that corresponds to that of adults.

So experience plays an important role in the development of concepts of death, as the results for the children under six show. It is interesting to note that in this study, as in those to follow, the focus is on so-called subconcepts or details of the total concept; these authors were trying to break the problem down into its individual aspects.

T. P. Reilly and collaborators (1981) studied the concepts of death of sixty children between the ages of five and ten with regard to age, factors related to cognitive development, and life experience with separations or death. They compared children from intact families with those who had suffered the loss of a close family member and with those who had experienced the separation and divorce of their parents. They found that most children older than six had ideas about the universality of death. Two-thirds of the five- and six-year-olds confirmed that they knew they would have to die someday. Their understanding of their own death was dependent on their level of cognitive development and their death-related experience. Their parents' separation, on the other hand, played no role. It is true, however, that this finding is contradicted by others (Sugar 1972; Zeligs 1974) who have equated the experience of separation (parents' divorce) with the experience of death. The work of Reilly and his collaborators shows that young children already know about death, and they pointed out explicitly that doctors need to be aware of that fact.

In 1984, Mark W. Speece and Sandor B. Brent published a survey of the empirical literature dealing with the development of death concepts in which they concentrated on three components: irreversibility, nonfunctionality, and universality. They concluded that the majority of healthy children between five and seven in modern urban-industrial societies develop an understanding of all three components. Speece and Brent cite many studies that document this early awareness (among others, thirteen dissertations from 1973 to 1978). This is also the age at which children migrate from preoperational to concrete-operational thinking, so it makes sense at the theoretical level, and it seems reasonable to see a connection between the two processes— the increase in understanding and the development of cognitive ability. Thus far, however, attempts to validate this connection empirically have not provided any unambiguous proof of this theory. This is discussed at length in the article by Speece and Brent. They wrote, "Piagetian theory is unlikely in principle to provide a complete picture of children's conceptions of death since it emphasizes the development of context-independent reasoning abilities."

They explained further that differing experiences with death affect the development of children's concepts. Children's experiences with death, which may include experiences with a death in their own environment as well as stories they have been told, are probably decisive for their understanding of death. If this is true, then in order to study children's concepts of death and cognitive development in general, we need a developmental model that takes account of both at the same time: the increase in knowledge *and* the development of context-independent reasoning ability.

In conclusion, Speece and Brent stated that younger children still believe in the reversibility of death to some extent, and they ascribed a multiplicity of life functions to inanimate objects. Often they still have the idea that death doesn't affect particular people, including themselves. On the other hand, the authors explained that most children at seven have developed concepts of death that include an understanding of the irreversibility, nonfunctionality, and universality of death.

The following year, another study was published dealing with subconcepts of children's concept of death (Hoffman and Strauss 1985). The subconcepts investigated were:

- death as the end of all functions
- the inevitability of death
- the irreversibility of death
- the cause (biological or physical)
- the universality of death

The details of the authors' complex investigation cannot be included here; it showed that the fundamental concept changes with age. The most important changes occur in three- and four-year-olds, which is why at five, children have correct answers to questions that refer to various subconcepts. Hoffman and Strauss discovered that the subconcepts followed a certain developmental sequence: the subconcept "universality" is followed by the three subconcepts "death as the end of all functions," "cause," and "irreversibility of death." At the end, an understanding of "the inevitability of death," obviously the most difficult for children to understand, develops. These findings show that the subconcepts do not develop all at once. Differing specific mechanisms may cause the subconcepts to develop at differing speeds. It is also possible, however, that the mechanisms are the same but the subconcepts differ in complexity, which would also lead to variation in development times.

R. Lansdown and G. Benjamin (1985) confirmed these findings in principle. One hundred and five healthy children were read a story about an old woman who had died and were then asked questions. These authors too studied the development of the various subconcepts and found that almost all eight- and nine-year-olds had developed a concept that was more or less complete. This was also true of approximately 60 percent of five-year-olds. Lansdown and Benjamin were able to determine that it is quite possible for five- or even four-year-olds who appear verbally competent to discuss death and its meaning with adults in a way that even today seems inconceivable to many adults.

Another study from the same year deals with the influence of age, animate objects, and the children's cultural and religious backgrounds on the subconcepts "irreversibility," "universality," and "inevitability" (Candy-Gibbs et al. 1985). Age clearly influenced acceptance of inevitability and universality as well as the children's understanding of their own death. It did not, however, influence their understanding of irreversibility, which was strongly influenced by their religious backgrounds (Southern Baptists' belief in life after death or Unitarians' belief in death as the end, for example). The same applied to the inevitability of death. The authors were not able to confirm a specific developmental sequence for the subconcepts.

An Israeli study from the same period, on the contrary, did find a sequential pattern in the development of subconcepts (Orbach et al. 1987). The authors investigated the ideas of 197 schoolchildren of various ages about several subconcepts (causality, finality, advanced age, irreversibility, and universality). They found that there were two developmental patterns depending on whether the death was human or animal. If it was a human being, the subconcepts were developed in the following order: advanced age, irreversibility, universality, finality, and causality. The subconcept of causality was obviously the most difficult for the children to understand. In the case of an animal's death, the order was somewhat different: irreversibility, universality, finality, advanced age, causality. The results were consistent in two independent studies. There were occasional deviations from the sequence described for the group as a whole.

There is a logical explanation for the sequence observed. The simplest subconcept is advanced age, which children can see and define. They learn first that old people are closest to death. The next step is the realization that death is irreversible. Children are most likely to learn this through the death of an animal, which is why this subconcept appears to be the easiest to understand in this context. Then they gradually learn that death is universal, something that is not directly visible or subject to experience; knowing about it depends on the information the children have gathered in the meantime. An understanding of the finite nature of life and the cessation of all functions that accompanies death is much more difficult to acquire. For that, an understanding of biological processes and their connection to the immobility characteristic of death is necessary. It is especially hard to understand that all feelings, thoughts, and consciousness end with death; this was already described at an earlier point (Kane 1979). Causality is clearly the most difficult concept for children; it requires a clear understanding of biological processes as well as the ability to think abstractly. White and collaborators (1978) believed that this subconcept is the most difficult to understand because it is a "scientific" concept. Such concepts are acquired through intuition and not "spontaneously" through experience. That the difference between younger and older animals is not obvious to children may explain why the subconcept of advanced age is difficult for them to understand in connection with animals' deaths.

At the end of the 1980s, Michael Stambrook and Kevin C. H. Parker (1987) summarized the knowledge accumulated up to that time in a survey article. They confirmed that a pattern in the development of children's concepts of death had become clear despite substantial variations in results. It appears that children progress from the idea of death as a transitory and reversible condition (like sleep and separation) to the idea of death as an internal and universal biological process. Many factors leading to conceptualization were described by various authors: experience with death, religious upbringing, living environment, cognitive and emotional development, mass media, and general sociocultural influences. Most interesting is what Stambrook and Parker wrote about age-dependent knowledge. They first cited I. Yalom (1980), who had reported that children under three already have some idea of the finality of death but deny it. Other authors (Kastenbaum and Costa 1977) had already expressed the same idea. Stambrook and Parker advised caution but stated that it seems obvious that many children can understand the finality of death under certain circumstances, for example due to the effect of the loss of a close family member; structured studies of children without this kind of experience do not reveal this kind of understanding (Nagy 1948; Lonetto 1980).

Stambrook and Parker further emphasized that children after the age of three and sometimes even earlier can have clear ideas about what death means. The literature, as I have described at length, shows substantial differences in the nature of these ideas. The authors observed that three- to five-year-old children are curious and want to find out about death even though they still imagine that it is reversible. Other authors had pointed out how important adults' statements are for children's concepts and that the emotional tone of these statements is registered just as clearly as their content (Speece and Brent 1984). Assessments in the literature of the role played by experience at this age are contradictory, as already mentioned. Stambrook and Parker did not take a clear position. Based on my own experience working in the hospital on a daily basis, I would place great importance on children's experience as well as on how parents handle this topic (how they talk with their children about it, for example).

There are also contradictory assessments in the literature about the ideas of six- to eight-year-olds concerning, for example, the finality of death. This may be because for many children from a religious background, life after death is conceivable, which of course contradicts the concept of finality. Stambrook and Parker think that sociocultural conditions have clearly changed in the course of past decades, which may have accelerated the ability to generate a realistic concept. In conclusion, the authors subscribed to the idea found in the literature that children at age nine have a clear idea of death—as a biological process that follows laws of nature. This concept of death differs from adults' way of thinking only in that it has a more pronounced influence on how children behave (Kastenbaum and Aisenberg 1972; Lonetto 1980). Other authors have also reported that thirteen- to sixteen-year-olds react to death with a greater emotional intensity than twelve-year-olds (Alexander and Adlerstein 1958). Myra Bluebond-Langner (1978) had determined earlier that adults' concepts differ from children's in style and language but not in content.

C. R. Cotton and L. M. Range (1990) studied children's concepts of death in relationship to the subconcepts "cognitive function," "age," "experience with death," "fear of death," and "hopelessness." In contrast to others (Reilly et al. 1983), they found a negative correlation between "experience with death" and an accurate concept of death, particularly as far as causality and inevitability were concerned. They saw the explanation for this in the religious backgrounds of the children they had studied. The children who gave religious answers ("Grandfather is with Jesus") scored noticeably lower in their concept of death than children without a religious background; in other words, their concept was less well developed. On the other hand, there was a pronounced positive correlation between cognitive maturity and concept. Conflict may arise with children who are cognitively more mature when adults try to convey a euphemistic image of death in their explanations that is contradicted by what the children know. So Cotton and Range too advocate an open and honest discussion with children. The authors found no apparent influence of either "fear of death" or "hopelessness" on the children's conceptual development; we have to consider, though, that the children in the study were not ill. What these authors have to say about sick children is addressed in the next chapter.

Alice Lazar and Judith Torney-Purta (1991) also studied the various subconcepts. They felt it was necessary to study them separately, since they develop separately. Thus comprehensive investigations of a concept of death are no longer appropriate. According to their findings, children in first and second grade understand the subconcepts "irreversibility" and "inevitability" first, but the development of one of these subconcepts is not dependent on the other. Children need an understanding of at least one of these two subconcepts in order to understand causality and the termination of life through death. Lazar and Torney-Purta also found a certain difference based on whether the death of an animal or a person was at issue. They concluded that most children think about death and develop an understanding of the relevant subconcepts even though many adults hesitate to broach the subject with them.

Conclusion

So everything began with Sigmund Freud, the founder of psychoanalysis, who at the beginning of the twentieth century was the first to think about children's viewpoints regarding death. He influenced many scientists who followed, both psychoanalysts and developmental psychologists, with his theoretical concepts. It was his unequivocal opinion that children know nothing about death and also don't think about it. His theories were viewed as guidelines by many scientists well into the second half of the twentieth century. Kastenbaum and Costa (1977) were the first to condemn this practice clearly, declaring that the uncritical acceptance of Freud's theories had stifled research in the field. Orthodox psychoanalytic theory is the reason for this effect; according to its tenets, ideas about death can only develop after the Oedipal phase, which can only occur if the Oedipus complex has been adequately resolved (Stambrook and Parker 1987). This implies that fears and thoughts about death are actually symbolic products or a manifestation of castration anxiety. It is true that analytically oriented theorists like Melanie Klein (1948) had already contradicted this theory by attributing central importance to concepts of death. But Freud's influence was so strong that not until the last quarter of the twentieth century were doubts about his theory considered seriously and new approaches sought.

To express it more simply: Freud fundamentally denied that young children were capable of attempting to come to terms with death. We can refer once more to his statements in *The Interpretation of Dreams,* where he stated that children know nothing of the horrors of decay and the terrors of eternal nothingness, so that fear of death is foreign to them. For many of his successors, and for pediatricians too, this meant that we do not need to discuss the topic of death with children. And only healthy children were actually studied. Until well into the second half of the twentieth century, terminally ill children were virtually never mentioned, as I discuss in the next chapter. At most, a researcher would occasionally suggest that the situation might be different for sick children, but no one pursued the issue or drew the logical conclusion that the appropriate studies should be done. For the adults—parents, teachers, or doctors—this idea was a great relief. Since death was a problem for many of them, they could ignore the topic with children in good conscience. From our viewpoint today, we would say that Freud didn't do children any favors with his theory. It is interesting to note, as I mentioned, that he added a section to the new edition of *The Interpretation of Dreams* in which, based on something he had observed, he formulated doubts about his own ideas in a preliminary way. This reversal was ignored by his successors, however, and he himself never revised his original position elsewhere, as far as I know.

Another scientist who studied the development of children and their concept of death intensively was the Swiss developmental psychologist Jean Piaget. He posited a multistage model of the development, postulating that children must master one stage before moving on to the next. And he believed that children don't reach a stage until the age of ten or even twelve at which they can begin to develop concepts of death similar to those of adults. According to Piaget, younger children are incapable of developing abstract concepts. This means that they cannot begin to understand death until their cognitive structures allow formal operational thinking, and that does not happen until puberty. For a long time, these theories formed the basis of scientific ideas about children's concepts and way of thinking, and they impeded a broader view. Many researchers who followed Piaget used his concept of stages as a point of departure and tried to corroborate it with additional data or possibly to modify it, but they never fundamentally questioned it. Finally, at the beginning of the 1970s, criticism began to be heard (Kastenbaum and Aisenberg 1972). In 1977, Kastenbaum and Costa pointed out that Freud's and Piaget's theories were often cited and used to support the idea that younger children are not capable of knowing much about death. They went so far as to ascribe a suffocating effect on research to the uncritical adoption of the concepts of Freud and Piaget, in my opinion a harsh but valid criticism of subsequent researchers.

Both Piaget and later Harry Stack Sullivan (1972) emphasized that the goal of personal human development is not just the ability to recognize one's own individuality; it is also the ability to develop relationships with other people. This makes it clear that the point here cannot be to achieve individuation and separation, as it is in many other theories. R. L. Selman and L. H. Schulz (1990) define the capability for autonomy as the capability of coordinating and connecting one's own wishes with those of another person. This viewpoint emphasizes the importance of relationships with others in child development, not the importance of separation. Autonomy is defined not as independence from other people but as the ability to recognize the need for other people and to establish a reciprocal relationship (Silvermann 2000). Piaget appears to have overlooked that at a very early age children can experience the loss of a relationship they have established as traumatic and can grieve about it.

Some of Piaget's successors tried to use the stages he had described in explaining developmental processes (Safier 1964; Koocher 1973; White et al. 1978; Speece and Brent 1984). Kastenbaum, for example (Kastenbaum and Aisenberg 1972), described how young children are quite capable of thinking about death despite the limitations imposed by their level of cognitive development. Others linked the concepts children use to understand life and death with the development of an understanding of animism. In research during this period, discussions of other factors that influence the development of children's concepts of death appear more frequently, so that the picture becomes more and more complex. Subconcepts are increasingly the subject of studies that describe and offer empirical evidence for a developmental sequence. Lazar and Torney-Purta (1991) later pointed out that we need to investigate the subconcepts individually in order to understand the children's concepts as a totality.

Seventy-five years after Freud's first deliberations, a picture of healthy children's concepts of death had developed that was based on substantial empirical data. Of course I did not cite all of the extensive scholarly literature but attempted to use key publications to trace the developments in research since Freud. Today we credit children with a much greater independent cognitive capacity. But the picture is still not clear and unambiguous. We more or less agree that death is understood at first as transitory and reversible. Later the idea of a universal biological process that is part of life and is linked to the end of bodily functions appears. We are still in disagreement about the age at which this occurs, but most researchers have recognized in the meantime that it must be much earlier than Piaget had thought. I am a pediatrician, and when all is said and done, I am interested in what sick children know. Therefore I think it is worth repeating that until the 1990s seriously ill or dying children are mentioned marginally or not at all in studies in the fields of developmental psychology and psychoanalysis. When they discuss influential factors, authors do admit that children's own experience with illness may be one of them. In an excellent survey, Stambrook and Parker (1987) wrote, "The evidence suggests that certain experiences (being terminally ill) can result in well developed understandings of death in very young children." Although these authors point to the fragmented nature of the picture and insist on more intensive research, it appears that at that point things came more or less to a standstill; few new and promising research results have appeared in the meantime.

It is astounding that Susan Carey, having reviewed the English-language literature of the past eighty years, wrote in her book *Conceptual Change in Childhood* (1985) that there is a solid literature about children's understanding of death. She stated that available research paints a surprisingly consistent picture based on the three stages described by Piaget and later by Nagy. My own account up to this point does not support this view at all. G. B. Mathews (1989) wrote in an article on the topic that no uniform ideas about children's thinking exist: "It would, indeed, be remarkable to find complete agreement on anything of importance in developmental psychology. It is especially noteworthy to find agreement on the difficult question of how we come to understand the ultimate threat to our own existence."

Mathews (1989) views his colleagues critically in his article. First, he describes the three stages as Carey (1985) defined them:

1. Children up to five years of age: Death, sleep, and departure are identical. The emotional effect comes through separation and aggression, death is neither final nor inevitable, and the dead person can come back. Cannot yet imagine a cause of death.
2. Children up to nine or ten years of age: The finality of death is understood, that is, that a person no longer exists after they die. The cause still comes only from outside, there is still no idea about what happens in the body as the result of the external event.
3. Children over nine or ten years of age: Death is understood as an inevitable biological process. In the case of the Hungarian children (Nagy 1948) who personified death in the second stage, the soul lives on after death. This religious idea is not very pronounced in American children. Ideas are more and more similar to those of adults.

Mathews explained that not everyone who has read this literature has come to the same conclusions as Carey. Speece and Brent (1984) came to entirely different conclusions, which Mathews obviously shares. And Mitchell too, in her useful book *The Child's Attitude to Death* (1966), pointed out that a maturation process is doubtless evident during the development of concepts of death. This maturation process differs from child to child, however, and is always dependent on the child's environment with its physical, mental, emotional, and social influences. Speece and Brent described three components of a concept of death: irreversibility, nonfunctionality, and universality. In their opinion, almost all studies show that children at age seven can understand and deal with all three.

Mathews emphasized that the concept Carey describes was based only on healthy children. He then turned to the book *The Private Worlds of Dying Children* by Bluebond-Langner (1978) about children terminally ill with leukemia; this important book will be considered in more detail in the next chapter during the discussion of sick children's concepts of death. Mathews too defines stages, five in this case, through which sick children reach an awareness of their situation. These stages are analogous to the stages defined by Piaget, but with a major difference. In Bluebond-Langner's concept there is also a step-by-step development from one stage to the next, but for her, chronological age plays absolutely no role. The children's experience is the determining factor. Many children remain at one stage for an entire year, others for only a week or two. She reported that many three- or four-year-olds with average intelligence knew more about their prognosis than some nine-year-olds who had not yet suffered a relapse of their leukemia, were in the hospital less often, and therefore had much less experience. When I discuss sick children's concepts of death in the next chapter, I will go in more detail into Mathew's reasoning, which shows that in fact the classical concept of development does not correspond to the ideas of children who are ill.

At the end of the 1980s, a new development was on the horizon. In the meantime, clinical medicine is more and more interested in how children deal with death. This interest now focuses on children's understanding of death and dying and no longer on whether severely ill and dying children are able to develop such an understanding. It is probably a result of doctors' increasing experience with dying children who succumb to the effects of their illness after a lengthy period. A public discussion about these children has also begun, not least because of the increasing interest in establishing hospices that were first intended for adults but are now also designed with children in mind.

CHAPTER NINE

Sick Children's Concepts of Death

Dying children frighten adults. Well into the nineteenth century, when it was still common for death to occur in public, in the presence of family and friends, the death of a child was, for adults, an occasion for sadness but not fear. A change began at the end of the century and continued into the twentieth century, as the topic of death became taboo in Western society. It became ever more difficult for adults to view death as a part of life. And, as I described earlier, death was increasingly banished from people's field of vision, taking place in the anonymity of a hospital rather than in a domestic environment. And people in the West may have been left dumbfounded by the horrors of two world wars in which people died in terrifying numbers. During the Second World War, at least, they often died far from home in military conflicts, but they also died in the cities during the innumerable nights of bombing or while fleeing at the end of the war. In these circumstances, as on the battlefield, people probably had to repress the thought of death in order to survive the horror.

Until the beginning of the twentieth century, children, especially infants and toddlers, often died quickly due to infectious diseases or nutritional disorders so that they had no time to confront the subject of death. Of course even then there were children with chronic diseases like tuberculosis or osteomyelitis (infection of the bone) that were usually untreatable. Such an illness could last months and sometimes even years. But parents probably seldom talked about death with the children. Doctors probably didn't even try to do so; after all, they were following the lead of the great doctor Christoph Wilhelm Hufeland, who lived from 1762 to 1836 and was a professor in Jena and Berlin. At the beginning of the nineteenth century, he declared, "He who names death, brings death." He was trying to say that even talking about the possibility that someone might die could precipitate death, because it would cause the patient to lose courage.

Medicine could do little to treat serious illnesses at that time because the causes of many diseases were still unknown. Doctors were often helpless to treat serious infections before the introduction of antibiotics. It was this helplessness that led to the general attitude that "the doctor should not take away the patient's hope." It was true that at the time, hope was often all the sick person had. I pointed out earlier that in Victorian literature, however, it was not at all assumed that you couldn't talk with children about death; by no means did the doctor "cause death if he mentioned it." And I have quoted Gottfried Keller (1972), who also painted a completely different picture in 1878 in an episode from *The Governor of Greifensee.*

In other words, during the first half of the twentieth century adults did not talk about death with children, just as they seldom talked about it with each other. In the last chapter, I discussed the fact that great thinkers like Freud, Piaget, and others had provided the basis for adults seeing no need to talk about dying and death with children. They asserted that young children know nothing about death and do not give it any thought. This led quickly to the idea that one should not talk about death with children. Even the highly respected educator and psychologist Eduard Spranger wrote in 1924 in his famous work *Psychologie des Jugendalters* (Psychology of adolescence), "Children do not understand death as such because they don't have the awareness to do so; they don't understand its meaning completely even when their own death is concerned."

For pediatricians, this and similar assertions were reason enough to base their concept of how to support seriously ill and dying children on this position. You didn't talk about death with children; you just answered their questions. But in your answers, you were to avoid the topics of death and dying absolutely. That was the explicit rule taught to all medical students well into the 1970s and 1980s; it was impressed on them, and that was also the approach their role models used. Of course, this approach was seen as valid in caring for adult patients as well as terminally ill children. For pediatricians, this was an explicit guideline, and they never questioned it; they were expected to follow it and were glad to do so. It had the advantage of allowing them to avoid any discussion of such a frightening topic with children. I too was taught this rule during my medical studies in the early 1960s, and when I began my training to become a pediatrician in 1971, nothing had changed. I mentioned earlier that as a student I already began to have my first misgivings about the validity of these ideas.

Doubts about this approach were slow to emerge in the medical community, however. It was probably the children with cancer who slowly conveyed to their doctors that things could be otherwise. This process dragged on throughout the last three decades of the twentieth century, and it is not over yet. This chapter will describe how pediatricians dealt with this topic at different times, and what their conclusions were. It will help us understand why it took so long for clear ideas about how children think to emerge, and how we as doctors should deal with this issue even though there is still no consensus. The final chapter of the book will address these issues in more detail. I have commented extensively elsewhere on what conduct is appropriate on a daily basis (Niethammer 2010).

That the literature discussed here relates for the most part to children and adolescents with cancer is not entirely due to my own involvement with such children. Oncology is simply the area in pediatric and adolescent medicine in which death hangs over the affected children and their parents from the very first day, although today fortunately only approximately one-fourth of children with cancer die of it. Things were still different at the beginning of the 1970s, when despite all attempts at therapy, only 5 to 10 percent of children with cancer survived. Staff in pediatric oncology were the first from any pediatric specialty forced to confront the death of children; it is true that the situation for children with cystic fibrosis, for example, was at one time not much different, since they died in the first or, at the latest, in the second decade of life. And children with inoperable cardiac defects or other congenital illnesses suffered a similar fate. Nevertheless, pediatric oncology is the source of most publications available to us today.

This field didn't develop into a separate subspecialty until the end of the 1960s. Until then, doctors were seldom able to cure children with leukemia and tumors unless they could surgically remove the malignant tumor completely, provided it had not yet metastasized. The early 1970s saw the first permanent therapeutic successes using chemotherapy to treat leukemia, and amazing advances were made in this area of pediatric medicine relatively quickly. Pediatricians who had entered this new subspecialty made up the majority of those closely involved in these developments. Previously, children whose chance for a cure was extremely poor were treated and cared for by pediatricians without any special training. Of course there were individual pediatricians—not specialists in today's sense of the word—who worked intensively with pediatric cancers, especially leukemia, very early on.

As far as I know, the first pediatrician to write about dying children, at least in Germany, was Bernhard de Rudder, professor of pediatric medicine in Frankfurt; it is true, however, that he was not one of the doctors most heavily involved in actually treating pediatric cancer. In 1950 he wrote in the *Deutsche Medizinische Wochenschrift* (German Medical Weekly), "There are still innumerable human lives extinguished year after year, still 'immature,' before their souls can experience a longing for death." This statement says two things: On the one hand, innumerable humans die during childhood, certainly an appalling balance sheet in the eyes of a pediatrician. On the other hand, it is comforting that children die in an "immature" condition. He explained what he meant by "immature" indirectly when he wrote that a child dies before its soul has any premonition of death. He called it a "longing for death," a psychoanalytical interpretation. This is obviously an unambiguous and reassuring fact in his eyes, and it implies that we do not need to talk about death with children. And pediatric medicine at the time conducted itself accordingly, in conformity with Freud's ideas.

We can easily identify this attitude in the context of later statements by de Rudder in his lectures. He spoke of levels of awareness and axioms in medicine, singling out two axioms in particular. He defined *axioms* as "the assumptions, statutes, or dogmas in every scientific field that are freely chosen, that are neither provable nor disprovable within the field, but once they have been chosen are in force and binding for everything that follows." One of the two axioms was the basic axiom of conduct for physicians. He defined the task of medicine: the healthy are to be kept healthy, the sick are to be made well, human life is to be preserved at any cost, and endangered life is to be saved. He added that the insistence on "preserving life at any cost" could also be referred to as the axiom of the primacy of life, his second axiom. The duty of attending the dying does not appear in this list. Perhaps it is not in line with the axiom of the primacy of life, whereby he insisted that people be cured even against their will. Thus the child who doesn't want to know anything about dying fits into his plan very well.

In 1955 the American pediatricians Julius B. Richmond and Harry A. Waisman were the first to publish a paper on the psychological aspects of caring for children with cancer. They confirmed that the death rate from infection, nutritional disorders, and metabolic disturbances had dwindled substantially so that cancers had become increasingly important for pediatricians. They saw that the percentage of children who would have to be admitted to a children's hospital and would die of cancer would continue to increase. With this in mind, the authors noted, it was amazing that so little had been written about this issue in pediatric medicine, although a paper on the same topic relating to adults had appeared a short time before. It is worth looking more carefully at a section of the original paper that deals with children's reaction to cancer:

> Children observed by us rarely manifested an overt concern about death. Even among adolescents, who intellectually may know much about cancer, the question concerning diagnosis and possibility of death usually was not raised as it often is by the adult patient. Our suspicion is that this does not reflect an awareness but rather represents an attempt at repression psychologically of the anxiety concerning death. For the occasional child who asked about his diagnosis, a simple descriptive statement was given without provision of a diagnostic label.
>
> In general, children seem to have reacted with an air of passive acceptance and resignation. Associated with this there often seemed to be an atmosphere of melancholia. Some of this may, of course, be the projection of the staff and parents rather than the child's feelings. Since the child's physical energy diminishes so significantly, it may be that much of the child's lack of emotional as well as physical response is due more to this factor than to psychological awareness of the diagnosis.
>
> During diagnostic and therapeutic procedures we have noted a tendency to greater passivity to the procedures than is present in normal children. Whether this is due in part to resignation or to the lack of physical energy is not known

at present. With the progress of the disease the passivity tends to become marked; it is not uncommon to observe children with extensive lesions and hemorrhage maintained entirely by parenteral fluid therapy without any significant protestations concerning its discomfort.

This is an amazing historical document, reflecting the state of most doctors' knowledge fifty years ago and demonstrating that there was no open communication at the time. Without any detailed discussion, the assumption is made that children don't want to know anything. In the rare instances when children do ask for information, they are lied to. Most of the article is devoted to the problems of parents, doctors, and members of the treatment team. The section on doctors is especially noteworthy. Richmond and Waisman pointed to the problem of "getting too close," which can lead to excessive involvement in the case, with the result that the patient receives more treatment than is appropriate because the doctor has lost his or her objectivity. They described the problems young doctors face when they have to care for too many cancer patients on a ward (more than three). In contrast to the usual situation when they aren't caring for cancer patients, these doctors are relieved when they can leave the oncology ward at the end of their rotation. We will see later that these problems were widespread and onerous for both doctors and nursing staff as long as their behavior toward the patients had not changed. And "getting too close" is still a problem, affecting young doctors more frequently but not limited to them.

In the following year the French pediatrician Jean Bernard and the French psychologist and psychoanalyst J. M. Alby (Bernard and Alby 1956) also published an article about the psychological problems triggered in children by leukemia. The authors reported that children as young as three or four are able to recognize the seriousness of their situation, although this is not often the case. They believed that we can assume that older children do have a clear understanding of their illness. Children react with subconscious defense mechanisms, and the fundamental form of defense is of course denial. Thus the threatening aspect of the illness is repressed. Bernard and Alby went on to say that this form of self-protection is often insufficient or superficial and no longer offers any real protection if the illness gets worse or at the end of life, during the transition to death.

Bernard and Alby supported their argument that we need to protect children from knowledge by citing the story of a thirteen-year-old boy who found out about his leukemia diagnosis and from that point on lived in fear and didn't want to go to sleep. In France, they reported, doctors talked openly at the children's bedsides about their illness and its consequences but tried to prevent adult patients from finding out about their diagnosis. It is clear that the French doctors felt that because children do not think about death, it could be discussed openly and without hesitation in front of them, an approach not viewed as appropriate with adult patients. Bernard and Alby wrote about how three- and four-year-olds listen intently when the doctors are talking. They put two and two together with regard to what is talked about in their proximity every day; they even think about the results of their examinations. It is fascinating to read how the children arrive at the understanding that they are lost. Some years earlier, H. Danon-Boileau, a doctor in Paris, had reported similar behavior in children with tuberculous meningitis. This disease was almost always fatal at the time, since effective medications for tuberculosis did not yet exist.

Bernard and Alby confirmed the resignation and passivity that the American doctors Richmond and Waisman had reported the previous year. They too described how the children's fear is concealed by their passivity; more important, they described the gradual transformation of the children's personalities. They noted that some children with leukemia are able at the age of four or five to express verbally that their end is approaching. Bernard and Alby expressly contradicted the ideas of Piaget, who had studied and written only about healthy children. They went on to say that fear of death becomes real for children with leukemia at the moment they understand—for a wide variety of reasons—the threat of death.

These observations are impressive, but their conclusion, viewed from today's perspective, is surprising. They wrote:

> Thus, it is one of the primary tasks of a doctor caring for leukemic children to prevent such fears from developing. Not only should the diagnosis not be revealed to the children, test results should never fall into their hands. Doctors' discussion, especially if they deal with therapies, have to take place in the children's absence. . . . During a hospital stay, we may sometimes have to mask the alert concern and affection with which we surround the child. In other words, it is very important that the little leukemia patient does not see or detect any differences between himself and his fellow patients in the room.

With this statement, the two French authors advocated an approach I was to experience as extremely stressful in the early 1970s: we were playing a part for the children who had cancer and for their fellow patients; we had to wear masks that were designed to hide our troubled faces. It became clear to us much later that we had succeeded only intermittently. This approach was extremely stressful, but it was what all of our colleagues in the hospital, as well as the sick children's parents, expected. After we pediatricians were allowed to stop this charade, after we started talking openly with the children, we finally realized what we had unnecessarily taken upon ourselves over the years with this approach, supposedly in the children's interest. How heavy this burden had really been for everyone involved became apparent through the relief we felt after it was over. Under these circumstances, we can see why Bernard and Alby devoted the second part of their article entirely to the problems of doctors and parents.

The approach to dealing with children with cancer proposed by Bernard and Alby was repeated almost ten years later by Walter Hitzig (1965) in Zurich. More than ten years after the French working group published their first paper, a follow-up was published (Alby and Alby 1967), in which the authors pointed to their observations of children and discussed studies that had been published in the meantime. Chief among them was one by Joel Vernick and Myron Karon (1965), who argued for absolute openness, including information about diagnosis; this article will be discussed at length later. The French authors, however, warned that openness is a double-edged sword, since it shifts the entire burden onto the patient and their families. Most of their article addresses problems of parents, siblings, and nurses. Parents should be allowed to stay in the hospital with their children—a demand that was surprising and far-sighted for the time, since visiting times had not yet been introduced in children's hospitals and parents were usually completely shut out.

It is striking that in 1967 the French authors Alby and Alby alluded to the problems of siblings, something not all doctors who treat children with cancer are aware of even today. On the whole, the article is empathetic and full of observations that were certainly new at the time. The conclusion they drew is all the more surprising—that despite having recognized how much children know, we should do everything we can to prevent this knowledge. They did have two important insights: that developmental psychologists' ideas worked out in studies of healthy children do not apply to children who are sick and that young children already know something about death.

In 1958 the book *Kind, Krankheit und Tod* (The child, illness, and death) by the developmental psychologist, educator, and philosopher Erich Stern was published in Germany. Having confirmed that the course of an illness is closely tied to life history, he wrote in the preface:

> Death shapes life too; it is not, as we may once have thought, an event that intervenes in life at a certain point in time; it determines life from the very beginning. Without death, without its constant threat, life would have a completely different character. Life would lack the restlessness, the feeling and awareness of the limits of existence, the irretrievability of time. Death sends its shadows well in advance in the form of fear of death, which is surely part of every life.
>
> What I am suggesting here is not only true for adults, it is true for children as well. Of course children's experiences are not the same as those of adults. All experiences are always determined by the general disposition of our personality, by its "totality," its "structure," and the structure of a child's personality is different from the personality of an adult. In addition, children lack many experiences that adults have had in the course of their lives and that determine their attitude.

Stern commented in his preface on the question of whether children think about death, the question that particularly concerns us here:

> Today many people still think that children are not concerned with the problem of death. That is true only conditionally, and above all only for children in the first years of life. But death soon attracts their attention, whether the occasion is the death of a close family member, overheard conversations, a first serious illness, or something else. We can see that a younger child usually doesn't yet really understand the meaning of death, that the child isn't familiar with death's finality and its irreversibility. Only gradually, as the child develops, does he form an idea of death that approaches reality more closely. And at the same time fear of death, which is not at all alien to children, emerges.

Stern, who had not studied children with cancer, expressed himself cautiously here, but it is clear that he had a different perspective—the perspective of someone who has cared for sick children. This factor differentiates him dramatically from all of the authors discussed in the previous chapter of this book who wrote about healthy children's concepts of death. Although he rejected the idea that young children "in general" are able to have an accurate idea of death, he nevertheless concluded that fear of death surfaces in the course of children's development. But for this to happen, a child has to be aware of death's meaning. At this point he could have cited as evidence Bernard and Alby's article (1956), which had appeared two years earlier, since they had already described how young children grapple with death.

In 1959 an article entitled "Sterben und Tod der Kinder" (Dying and the death of children) by Carl-Gottlieb Bennholdt-Thomsen, professor of pediatric medicine in Cologne, appeared in the *Deutsche Medizinische Wochenschrift*. The article was reprinted unaltered in 1979 in *Leben und Sterben in den Augen eines Kindes* (Living and dying in the eyes of a child), edited by Munich pediatrician Theodor Hellbrügge. Bennholdt-Thomsen wrote that no pediatrician is spared the experience of children's dying and their death. He wondered how children deal with their fear of dying and death, and how they behave when fear becomes unavoidable reality, in other words, when they die.

To answer this question, Bennholdt-Thomsen compiled case histories from his hospital reported to him by colleagues, so the observations are not his own. I briefly describe two of these cases here. The first is a boy just turned fifteen who remained suspicious about the intentionally false diagnosis that was reported to him. Using a different name, he phoned the laboratory and asked about his blood count, probably because he had picked up the word *leukemia* during a doctor's visit. Soon afterward, staff left a falsified medical report in his room "by mistake." The boy never talked about his prognosis, but during his last night he asked the nurse whether he would die during the night. The second case was a child just turned three with a brain tumor, who said before his bedtime prayer that "he would soon be with the angels too."

Bennholdt-Thomsen assumed that in many cases the children had a premonition of their imminent death. And none of the children, as he explicitly emphasizes, was wrong. It was the isolation of the dying children that he obviously found depressing. His conclusions remain general, yet they go beyond what his American and French colleagues had written. In his conclusion, he wrote that doctors' behavior in the face of the primacy of death is determined by the "how" of dying, and that possibly a better understanding of the "how" might lead to better palliative care. With this statement, he was pointing doctors at the time toward the correct approach, but it would be a long time until doctors finally understood the "how" adequately.

The German pediatrician Johannes Oehme, who had begun studying the treatment of children with leukemia in the 1950s, cited Bennholdt-Thomsen's work in a survey article on the hospital and therapy of acute leukemia in children published in 1960. He added nothing further, however, and did not develop any ideas for future improvements (Oehme 1958, 1960). He did take note of Bennholdt-Thomsen's work, at least, but he had at best a vague suspicion of its importance for children with leukemia.

In 1960, articles by two American authors appeared about a hospital program in which they inaugurated the participation of parents in the care of their children with cancer (Knudson and Natterson 1960; Natterson and Knudson 1960). They also wrote about their observations of fear of death in both children and mothers. They described how children over ten are often just as fearful as younger children. However, their fears are not alleviated by their mother's presence to the same extent. These older children think about their future and sometimes ask whether they will get well again or whether they are dying. They withdraw and are anxious and depressed. This is particularly the case when other children on the ward die. Knudson and Natterson saw sufficient reason to assume that children know about other children's deaths, even if they were not informed.

It is interesting to note that the children seldom ask about the deceased. The authors also pointed to the fears of younger children, which they tend to express through drawings and stories. Their essential finding is that children's fear goes through a maturation process. In children under six, separation anxiety is most prominent; in children from six to ten, it is the fear of physical injury; and in children over ten, it is the fear of death. Knudson and Natterson perceived a general agreement with Nagy's (1948) description of concepts of death in healthy children. The two authors said little about their own dealings with the children's anxieties. They mentioned that most children seem satisfied with minimal explanations for the absence of a deceased child. The exceptions are children who have evidence that the proffered explanations aren't correct or children who are generally mistrustful. In these cases, hospital staff did not deny that a death had occurred.

In an article by a prominent German pediatric oncologist (Hertl 1961) about experiences with parents of children with leukemia, the work by Bernard and Alby (1956) is cited without comment. Children's problems are hardly mentioned; the one exception is the remarkable suggestion that at the end of a consultation with parents, the doctor should try to engage the child in a lively conversation or a game, thus making it easier for the parents to return to a comfortable interaction. Didn't the doctors see that this was impossible for the parents, since they had almost certainly been crying in despair? And today we know that children usually see through this kind of parental behavior.

In 1963, James Morrissey, an American, described observations of fifty children with cancer in an attempt to investigate their adaptation to the deadly disease. The author, a social worker and not a doctor, summarized the information about the children that he had received from the treatment team as follows: Approximately half the children showed indications of anxiety during their entire hospital stay; the two- and three-year-old children, for whom support and comfort from their mothers were central, were the exception. The children communicated their anxiety in very different ways. Younger children expressed it in words or actions, and older children tended to become depressed. Parents can help the children adapt, but this doesn't always happen. About a third of the children speculated about the seriousness of their illness. This is a result of their fear of death or at least leads to it, in Morrissey's opinion. Fear of death had been observed only in older children, but here one three-year-old showed definite signs. The intensity of the anxiety reflects how well the children adapted to the situation. It is surprising that Morrissey was able to recognize fear of death in a relatively large percentage of the children based solely on the observations reported by the treatment team.

In the United States, an article by Joel Vernick and Myron Karon (1965) was published under the noteworthy title "Who's Afraid of Death on a Leukemia Ward?" Vernick was a social worker who was always in attendance on a leukemia ward and had close contact with the fifty-one children between nine and twenty-one years of age. All had been admitted to the hospital with acute leukemia. The interviews he conducted with the children concentrated on events as they unfolded. The goal was to gather clinical experience and offer psychological help at the same time if problems arose. What he and Karon, a pediatrician, presented in the article is unusual for the time. Every child on the ward knew when another child had died because they learned quickly how to interpret the changes associated with a death. Whenever a child was moved to a single room during the terminal phase, the other children passed by the room at least once a day to sneak a peek. And they asked what had happened to a child who had died. In the beginning, in order to protect the child asking the question from bad news, staff tended to say that the child had been transferred to another ward. It soon became apparent, however, that none of the children believed this subterfuge. The team had a discussion after one boy fiercely resisted being transferred to another ward due to space limitations. After a furious struggle, he had shouted that he didn't want to go to the place where children died. He had observed that none of the children who were transferred ever returned.

From then on, the team members gave honest answers to questions about children who had died—in 1965! They recognized that the subterfuges were preventing the development of a supportive relationship between the children and themselves. They understood that children fall silent when they accept lies outwardly but in reality feel abandoned with their fears. And this happens exactly at the point when children most need support. In their articles, Knudson and Natterson showed that children sometimes don't ask questions. Adults have to take the initiative in talking about death, since they have greater emotional strength (Knudson and Natterson 1960; Natterson and Knudson 1960). We can approach a child and tell them that another child has died because he or she was very ill. This way children perceive that team members can talk calmly about things they themselves find disturbing. A short time later, Emma Plank, a specialist in therapeutic education (1969), confirmed the soundness of this approach. Even very sick children benefit when team members recognize their situation and sympathize. In contrast to earlier reports in which children responded to this kind of information with a passive and resigned attitude (Richmond and Waisman 1955), Vernick and Karon and Plank observed that every child who lies in bed severely ill is thinking about death and hoping that someone will help him or her talk about it.

Vernick and Karon reported that they informed all children over age nine, and sometimes younger children, of their diagnosis. Each of the children accepted the explanations about the chronic nature of their illness without a strong reaction. Often the children were relieved, because their parents had already indicated how serious the illness was through their behavior, no matter how hard they tried not to. The authors went even further, making sure that the rest of the family, in particular siblings, were informed. Otherwise, misunderstandings and jealousy might develop and prevent the family from mobilizing its strength. Vernick and Karon also saw this procedure as the best way to protect children from hearing their diagnosis through their friends, since such information usually gets around.

They also emphasized how important it is to explain to children why certain procedures are necessary (a liver biopsy, for example) and to get their consent. This too was usually not talked about at the time; it was the parents who had to give consent. You did with the children whatever you thought was right and necessary. Two years earlier, the social worker James Morrissey (1963) had reported, based on observations of the treatment team, that only about 30 percent of the children gave any indication that they were afraid of death. But Vernick and Karon showed that observation alone can never provide clear results; only an active process can do justice to children's needs. None of the children they approached in this way withdrew permanently. In the course of their observations the two authors became increasingly certain that the "protective" approach recommended by others was incorrect. In conclusion, they answered the question posed in the title of the article as follows: "Who's afraid of death on a leukemia ward? Everyone—and the resolution of this fear is everyone's problem."

This article, published more than forty years ago, did not represent the spirit of the time at all. Vernick and Karon had already worked out the principal aspects of care for dying children. It is hard to believe that this work didn't immediately become the guideline for medical conduct, but instead it was quickly forgotten. It was cited repeatedly, but its contents probably frightened readers. The protective approach recommended by prominent representatives of the field catered much better to the ideas and anxieties of doctors, so an open approach could not gain acceptance at that time. This is strikingly conveyed in an editorial in the journal in which the article was published; it was written by two prominent pediatricians who also had experience with treating children with leukemia (Agranoff and Mauer 1965).

Joseph H. Agranoff and Alvin M. Mauer emphasized that children seldom ask questions and that the consequences of revealing a diagnosis can be highly problematic. The authors were working under unusual conditions that don't allow for generalization, since they were working on a ward where there were exclusively children with leukemia. In most other hospitals, the children with cancer would not be housed on a single ward. Agranoff and Mauer's curious counterargument was that increasingly subjective reports and comments about the illness, which were being printed in the lay press, were not desirable reading material for the children and their parents, who needed to be protected from them. They did not explain what happened to the children who somehow learned about their diagnosis, who were not in a position to talk with anyone if the information frightened them. Many years would pass before the majority of pediatric oncologists would accept the correctness of Vernick and Karon's concept and begin to act accordingly. The article's publication in 1965 instigated a discussion of this approach, which often included restrictive or even dismissive arguments, and this discussion has lasted until quite recently, as we will see.

The American pediatrician Morris Green (1967), in his article in *Pediatrics,* the most prominent American journal in the field, also advocated being honest when children ask about a child who has died. Otherwise, he repeated the developmental concepts that don't admit to children knowing about death until after puberty, although he did recognize that younger children also possess concepts of some kind. He emphasized that children seldom ask if they are dying and that we should never answer this question in the affirmative. Green was clearly very uncertain, since he seemed to suspect that children do know when they are dying and that they do possess a concept of death.

Two years later, an article by an American group was published in the renowned *New England Journal of Medicine* (Binger et al. 1969). They summarized the contents of interviews with twenty parents whose children had died of leukemia. Most of the children who were older than four had made it clear to their parents that they realized how serious their illness was, although no one had told them the diagnosis. They even sensed that death was imminent. Fourteen of the parents tried everything to shield their child from the diagnosis. The children who knew about their diagnosis also protected their parents if they realized that their parents didn't want to talk about it. The authors noted that these were the loneliest children of all.

It is also interesting to read their reports about two teenagers who had been told that their illness was incurable. Both families reported that their subsequent relationship to their children became closer than ever before. They suspected that it was the open communication that had brought this about. Binger and associates believed that it is a serious mistake to assume that children over five are not aware of the seriousness of their illness and of the possibility that they may die. The question is not whether we say something to the children but how we say it. It is surprising that the authors arrived at this conclusion through interviews alone; the conversations with the parents must have been intensive. There are statements from the same period by other authors who are sure that young children know about their own death and can express this knowledge (Kliman 1968).

Pediatric surgeon C. Everett Koop also published an article in 1969 about caring for dying children and their families. In this article, which is well worth reading, he reflected on a broad spectrum of physician behavior in connection with seriously ill and dying children. He also included a short passage about interacting with a dying child. He began by saying that in his assessment, honesty is probably the best approach in such interactions. In the next sentence, he wrote that children seldom make inquiries—an argument familiar from other authors. He closed with the thoughtful words: "I am convinced that many more children have known they were dying than shared that information with me. Some knew it and kept it from their family; with a few I have discussed death, at their request. I have not seen a child upset by this. With many, I have talked about close calls—after the fact. One can only gently feel his way along this uncharted path and be guided by the child." We can see from his choice of words that Koop was not entirely sure his thinking is correct, probably in part because it contradicted the established medical orthodoxy of that time.

What was the situation in the German-speaking countries at the time? P. Sachtleben (1970), a pediatrician in the town of Homburg, wrote in the *Monatsschrift für Kinderheilkunde* (Monthly Journal of Pediatrics) about what he had learned working with E. E. Osgood (1963) in Portland, Oregon, caring for a large number of leukemia patients. He argued for open communication with children; in his experience they feel freer and sometimes happier if nothing terrible is concealed from them. At the same time, he emphasized that until puberty, children do not have a clear concept of death and that dying children often have no perceptible fear of death. To be sure, he quoted an American study from 1952 by W. Alvarez about dying adults. In addition, he referred to the French studies discussed earlier, so we get the impression that he had few experiences of his own to draw on.

The same journal published a lecture by Hamburg pediatrician Karl-Heinz Schäfer (1972) two years later asking whether we must or should tell children the whole truth. In the first part of his lecture, he showed pictures painted by children in which fear of death was evident. Then he answered his own question by saying that in his experience, we should avoid telling the truth, because children "as a general rule are not in a position to process this reality rationally." Doctors should not destroy children's naiveté by force even in crisis situations in their lives. Nevertheless, we should not simply respond with an untruth if an older child or adolescent asks a precise question. But that—a precise question—was very rare, in his experience. He quoted the Protestant theologian and ethicist Helmut Thielecke from his book *Theologische Ethik* (Theological ethics) in which he described the doctor's position between the obligation to protect and the obligation to tell the truth:

"Whether the doctor lies or not is not dependent on whether he denies the situation or admits it straightforwardly at the moment . . . it depends on whether he views the potential denial as the first or preliminary phase of the process toward truth into which . . . he is determined to lead the invalid." Schäfer added that we will not usually have to tell children the truth about their illness. He hesitated even about telling the truth to parents. He reported that he once waited as long as seven weeks to tell parents that their child had leukemia because they didn't ask (!).

Likewise, psychologist Annemarie Wunnerlich published her useful book *Zur Psychologie der ausweglosen Situation* (On the psychology of the hopeless situation) in 1972; in it, she reported on children she had cared for in the children's hospital in Zurich who were ill with or dying from leukemia. She gave a striking portrayal of the children's behavior and discussed their care at length. Finally she came to the crucial question of whether children should be told the truth about their illness. She pointed out that this issue had been discussed repeatedly in the American literature. She wrote that in her opinion, children can only be confronted with the truth if they have dependable help and support in working through all their problems and every new piece of information they receive. This sentence should be emphasized, since even today many doctors have not yet realized that we cannot leave patients alone with negative messages and information. Wunnerlich wrote further that this kind of help "may be available in a treatment center to a certain extent." However, children with leukemia were beginning to live much longer at the time and were returning home to their normal environment more often; today this is common practice. In this situation, Wunnerlich thought that being aware of the probable outcome may create an unreasonable burden.

Wunnerlich's comments, in which she stated that it is obvious that complete secrecy is not a possibility, express incredible ambivalence. She remarked that it is perfectly possible to talk with children about their illness and the problems that result without confusing and frightening them with the fact that death is unavoidable. On the other hand, she was convinced that many children sense a great deal during the course of their illness. But then she emphasized—she viewed this as very important—that "many children never associate their serious illness directly with their own death. Instead, their fear results at least in part from the fear felt by adults, who cannot sustain a natural and for the most part honest relationship with the sick child without talking with him about the reason—namely the illness—for the fear they are both feeling."

These are the comments of a psychologist who is certainly intelligent and dedicated, and they describe the problem that many people struggle with when they have to care for dying children. Her book demonstrates clearly that she understood the children's problems. But it is hard for us today to relate to the conclusions she drew. How can we be honest with seriously ill children for the most part without talking about death? How can we gain children's trust if we evade the crucial point, as Wunnerlich suggested? She didn't respond to these questions, either because she didn't recognize the problem that is generated by her suggestions on how to behave, or, more likely, because she had no answer. She seemed to feel uneasy, however, since it would otherwise be hard to understand why she emphasized so strongly that most children do not connect their illness with death. If you are satisfied that this is the case, then the approach she suggested has a certain inner logic, but that does not make it correct.

In her closing chapter, in which Wunnerlich spelled out the practical implications for psychology, she made many good, noteworthy suggestions for providing support to parents and then discussed the children once more. She even quoted the American articles (Natterson and Knudson 1960; Vernick and Karon 1965) in which the authors wrote that we have to stop hoping to protect children from the truth. In Wunnerlich's opinion, this would work only in a treatment center for children with leukemia. In Europe, children would seldom be admitted to the hospital, and if they were, then they would be treated together with other sick children on the same ward. This would enable the children to lead a life that was normal for the most part, and they would be less oppressed by their illness. The pediatricians cited earlier from German-speaking countries who were involved in caring for children with leukemia (Schäfer, Oehme, Hertl, Hitzig) confirmed Wunnerlich's views. Her book is otherwise very interesting, but it is too bad that she shied away from the final step that would have helped many children at the time. We know now that a "life that is normal for the most part" is an illusion.

Anna Freud, whose father was the originator of psychoanalysis, dealt with the same topic (Freud and Bergmann 1972). She and her coauthor T. Bergmann wrote: "We don't know what is the right thing to do when we find ourselves faced with the task of preparing a child for death, whether it be the death of a fellow patient or his own death. For children, death means little more than the idea of being away, of having disappeared." Repeating the comment her father made almost seventy years earlier she denied that children have an understanding of death. This fact is astounding, considering that in England after the war she worked intensively with children who had lost their parents in air raids. She must have been so deeply entrenched in psychoanalytic developmental concepts that for her, the children's experience didn't appear to play a fundamental role.

In 1971 *Working with Children in Hospitals* by Emma Plank, a specialist in therapeutic education, was published in the United States (published in 1973 in Germany under the title *Hilfen für Kinder im Krankenhaus*). One chapter in this worthwhile book has the title "If Death Occurs on a Children's Ward." Plank reported on her experiences with dying children but did not really address the issue of the development of concepts of death. She believed that a child's death on the ward is of great importance for the other children, even though this may not be obvious to an observer. She went into detail about the fact that it is wrong to hide such an event from the other children. She wrote: "Children always observe and sense situations which adults wish and believe they did not see. Invariably they sense the strained and sinister, and if not helped to clarify what they think happened, the adults' silence may increase their fears in fantasy, rather than spare them sorrow."

Plank described the children's fear, which can be overwhelming if we fail to see that children need affirmation of themselves and their future. From her observations, children's reactions to death are quite varied. She too argued for honesty, but we can see that she was ambivalent, as were other authors of that period. Although she was convinced that even young children "know," she wrote: "When a young child who may conceivably die during hospitalization brings up the question of the possibility of his own death, we reassure him with great conviction and help the child in his attempts to deny the possibility. We would never try to prepare a child for his own death; however, we would facilitate his expression of thoughts and anxieties."

Here Plank was actually rejecting the open provision of information she had earlier demanded. But near the end of the chapter, she wrote: "How to help older terminally ill children with their feelings is an especially difficult question. They generally know that they are 'not supposed to know,' they tend to deny the severity of their illness so as to be able to live with it, and yet they desperately want our honesty." And later she elaborated: "Children build their defenses to protect themselves from too much pain, but they also want to know the truth. . . . Denial may still occur and should be left undisturbed, as it serves a protective function. The important thing is that the child know that he can trust the adults' honesty and ask questions when he wants to."

Plank, like Wunnerlich before her, exhibited a strange back and forth between demanding honesty and taking the decisive step toward complete openness. How can children depend on adults' honesty if their answers constantly evade the children's questions? Nevertheless, her clear statement that even very young children know about death and that we have to talk with them about it is important in this context.

Another study from the same year looked at fifty children between the ages of six and ten; in 1971 they had been admitted to an American children's hospital due to leukemia or a chronic disease that was not life-threatening (Spinetta et al. 1973). At that time, a leukemia diagnosis was still a death sentence. The authors reported that the children with leukemia were much more bothered by anxieties than the children in the control group. They obviously realized how serious the situation was without talking openly about it. The authors' statement that the children "obviously realize the seriousness of the situation" is surprising, since Myron Karon was one of the coauthors, and he had published the important paper in 1965 with Vernick (Vernick and Karon 1965) in which they reported unambiguously that children were definitely aware.

John Spinetta and his collaborators explained that it is just a question of semantics whether we label the nonconceptual fear of one's own terminal illness "fear of death." Spinetta published a literature survey the following year on reports that contradicted each other as to whether children with life-threatening illnesses are aware of the fact or not (Spinetta 1974). He and Lorrie J. Maloney then published a further study, this time about children with leukemia who were treated as outpatients (Spinetta and Maloney 1975). They assumed their findings would be comparable to those in the preliminary study, and in fact the children who lived at home were no different from those who had been treated as inpatients from the very beginning. Their anxiety did increase if visits to the outpatient clinic occurred with greater frequency or if they had to be admitted to the hospital. So it was not the hospital that triggered their anxiety but the illness itself.

German psychologist Wolfgang Larbig described the situation of terminally ill children in the hospital (Larbig 1974). He discussed the concepts of developmental psychologists in detail and mentioned that children's experience can definitely play a role in the development of their concepts. He went into great detail about the difficulties children experience due to being shielded from the experience of death, because death is a taboo subject in society today and medicine is increasingly aiming for perfection. The isolation of the dying inhibits the development of concepts, and it prevents a more rational attitude toward death on the part of dying children, their families, and the hospital staff. According to Larbig, this can lead to conflict-laden tensions within the hospital. He reported in detail about a conference on the scope of duties of the psychosocial professions in hospitals in which children die. The orientation of the discussion was clearly technical; he wrote nothing at all about the children themselves or concepts that might be helpful to them.

Larbig's work demonstrates that the discussion in Germany at the time clearly lagged behind the international one. This is also reflected in the work of pediatrician Ottheinz Braun (1976), who was one of the first in Germany to abolish visiting times in the children's hospital and permit parents to be with their children all the time. In a journal directed at established pediatricians, he described the international discussion in detail and cited the available literature. Unfortunately he didn't take the next step and at least tentatively develop some clear ideas about what course of action doctors should pursue. Here again we see the ambivalence of the pediatrician who has experience but doesn't really have confidence in it. And at the time, the scientific literature was in fact contradictory. R. Zeligs, an American, wrote in his 1974 book about children's experience with death that a six-year-old does understand the irreversibility and inevitability of death.

I would like to mention one other book by a non-physician, *L'enfant et la mort. Les enfants malades parlent de la mort: Problèmes de la clinique du deuil* (The child and death. Sick children talk about death: Problems in grief therapy) by the Parisian psychoanalyst Ginette Raimbault, which was published in France in 1975 and in German translation in 1980. She worked in a children's hospital with severely ill and dying children who were suffering primarily from renal failure. She reported in detail the experiences she had with various children, told their stories memorably, and often reproduced what was said word for word. Raimbault was not seeking concepts or theories; she let the children speak for themselves. I quote her here, because no paraphrase could convey her meaning as well. The introduction is the only chapter in which Raimbault gave a general description of her own ideas about how children think, always against a background of experiences with individual children. She quoted, for example, an eleven-year-old girl with a brain tumor who complains about adults' silence: "They don't tell me anything, but I know I have a tumor. People die. . . . Children die, I'll die too."

Another quotation from the book:

> If we emphasized the sick children's words, it is because we intend from the start to castigate the misconceptions and self-delusion that adults put up as a protective barrier: between the child and death, but in reality between death and themselves. Children can think these words. But they can only be heard and absorbed by those, whether children or adults, who permit these thoughts to get through to them. If children don't encounter anyone who can put themselves in their place, if they encounter only lies and silence, then they themselves will be silent. But, some will argue, children don't know what death is. Even if they talk about it, they don't have the same idea of death. And we? Who would claim to know what death is? Children have no need for philosophical concepts to confront death, see it, think about it, imagine it, accept it, reject it.

A few pages later, she writes:

> We cannot determine an age-appropriate concept of death, not based on the knowledge that children express about their future death, not based on the vague fear of death that seems to be their fate, not in the ideas they have about it, not in the meanings they attach to it. This may be the difference between a child who is physically healthy and one who is physically ill, between a child who has never experienced the death of a person close to him and one whose relationships with others have been disrupted. Such a child, like every other human being, has been prompted to think about the events experienced—illness, death—that changed his relationship to himself, his body, and to others. This inevitable thought process appears to lead children to the same ideas, conclusions and reasoning as adults.

In Raimbault's opinion, all children have a clear knowledge of their future death, which is always related to their illness and which is part of their illness. She also emphasized that this clearsightedness cannot prevent all defense mechanisms against the idea of death (denial, isolation, projection, deferral, mastery, humor).

It is impressive how this psychoanalyst, reporting about her personal experiences with seriously ill and dying children and adolescents, simply jettisoned the efforts and results of her colleagues during the first eight decades of the twentieth century to determine age-appropriate concepts of death held by children. She did so with the terse comment that these concepts aren't valid for sick children and may not be the right approach for healthy children either. She went much further than her Swiss colleague Wunnerlich several years earlier; nothing remains of the ambivalence we saw there. It is unfortunate that Raimbault documented many observations in her book but almost never commented on what could have been done in any individual case or what actions she took. So the book is theoretical and analytical, or, to be more precise, it is a book that can be recommended to any reader who would like to know but has little opportunity to observe how children think, speak, and behave in a life-threatening situation. But the reader will learn little about how we should actually behave in interactions with such children.

In the same year, the oncologists at the Oklahoma Children's Memorial Hospital published a study that created something of a sensation about what they called a final-stage conference (Nitschke et al. 1977). Twenty children with cancer and their parents were told that their cancer could not be cured with conventional treatments. The authors offered an experimental therapy. Three of the children were six or seven years old; these children also knew about their situation and made decisions like the older children did. I mention this study at this point because the authors clearly assumed that the children had already given thought to death. I return to this article in more detail in the chapter on children's participation in making decisions in chapter 11.

A year later, the German psychologist G. Wolff (1978) published an article with the title "Warum schweigen die krebskranken Kinder?" (Why do children with cancer keep silent?). He confirmed that many recent authors agree that most sick children know by the age of four or five how threatening their illness is (he cites Binger et al., Braun, Green, Spinetta, and Waechter). He also agreed that children send many indirect and nonverbal signals, and he asked why sick children talk so little about their feelings of fear and foreboding and about death and dying—in other words, why are they silent? Wolff concluded that it isn't the children's ignorance that keeps them silent; the reason lies with the adults around them. The silence shows the effectiveness of taboos and anxieties. Silence and repression may sometimes be helpful in maintaining psychological balance, but in most cases it means a silent curtailment of possibilities for life and experience. For this reason, Wolff insisted on better psychological support for the children, although he offered no definite guidelines for action. In an article published a year later under the title

"Was wissen denn schon die Kinder?" (1979; What do children know, after all?), he discussed the reasons that caregivers are silent. For him, it was no longer a question of whether or not the children "know."

In 1978, an interesting book by anthropologist Myra Bluebond-Langner was published in the United States. She studied children three to nine years old who had cancer, noting that previous studies have been contradictory. She devoted one chapter to describing what terminally ill children know about the world. It is impressive how well she described the behavior of these and other children in the hospital. The children understand what test results mean for them, what the therapy consists of; they know about side effects, and they understand the prognostic significance of a relapse. Bluebond-Langner dealt extensively with the question of how children gain their experience, and she made it clear that children's concepts of death are always the result of a developmental process; no child has a finished concept ready right off the bat. The author described this development in children with leukemia in five stages:

- Stage 1: The child understands that a serious illness is involved.
- Stage 2: The child learns the names and side effects of medications.
- Stage 3: The child comprehends the goal of treatment and what procedures are necessary.
- Stage 4: The child learns that the illness is a series of relapses and remissions (without death).
- Stage 5: The child knows that the illness will be fatal at some point in time.

She described the gain in experience with each of the stages. All of this applies to this type of illness, and the stages are different for different illnesses. Of course these stages are not exactly the same in all children, but they are similar. Bluebond-Langner described the developmental stages of the children's self-concept in parallel to this increasing experience:

0. healthy
1. seriously ill
2. seriously ill, but will get better
3. always ill, but will get better
4. always ill, and will never get better
5. dying

In Stage 5 of this concept, all children know that they are dying, and most comment about it. Bluebond-Langner reported that these comments are usually brief. She gave many examples, noting that many of these statements are both dramatic and inadequate. A five-year-old boy, for example, who is lying on his back in an uncomfortable position, is asked whether he would like to be turned over. "No," he answers, "I'm practicing for my coffin." Bluebond-Langner reported that the children are aware that their lives are finite, and therefore they don't want to waste any time. She also believed that children at this stage no longer make any plans for the future. I myself have often had a different experience, that children are able to make long-term plans despite knowing that they will die soon. The coexistence of two "real worlds," a phenomenon that we can also observe in adults, will be discussed later.

In a chapter on "Knowing and Concealing," Bluebond-Langner asked the same question that had occupied Wolff the year before: If all the children know they are dying, why don't they talk about it, and why do they try to conceal their knowledge? She referred to an idea of "knowing" that Glaser and Strauss (1965) had defined in a book on the subject. They wrote that we can understand the attitude of the dying best in the framework of a phenomenon they call "awareness context." Glaser and Strauss defined "awareness context" as follows: It is "what *each* interacting person knows of the patient's defined status, along with his recognition of the others' awarenesses of his own definition. . . . It is the context within which these people interact while taking cognizance of it." The authors identified four types of awareness that apply here:

1. Closed awareness: The patient does not recognize that he will die soon, while all others are aware of it.
2. Suspicion awareness: The patient suspects that others are aware of something. He or she tries to either confirm this suspicion or to view it as unfounded.
3. Mutual pretense: Both sides are aware that the patient is dying but behave as if the opposite were the case. They agree, so to speak, on the idea that the patient will live on.
4. Open awareness: Both sides know that the patient is dying and act in a relatively open manner.

Glaser and Strauss argued that it is important to understand the context in which the awareness occurs because of the effect on the behavior of everyone—the patient, the family, and the treatment team. People manage their conversations and actions according to who knows what and with what level of certainty. The prevailing context can only be sustained if everyone sticks to it. If the current context is closed awareness, for example, and one of the people involved activates the patient's suspicion that he is dying, then the context moves to the next stage or the one after that. Reciprocal deception is a delicately balanced situation with an abundance of rules, and it inevitably collapses, leaving open awareness as the unavoidable consequence.

This is the context for Bluebond-Langner's conclusion that the conditions for practicing reciprocal deception in the case of children are there from the start—before the diagnosis is really clear. The team is eager to keep the information away from the patient, to prevent leaks, and to plug them quickly if they occur. Children's attempts to learn the truth are blocked. Members of the treatment team and parents make it clear that they are not prepared to answer questions honestly. Although the children know everything, Bluebond-Langner believed they never reach the context of open awareness. She wrote, "We have established that the children with leukemia were aware of their prognosis, that they concealed this awareness from others, and we know how they did so." In closing, she stated, "We have not established *why* they concealed their awareness, and why others concealed their awareness from them."

Her answer to this question is different from that of other authors. Making a taboo of death is not the reason for these secrets. Instead, this approach allows each person to assume the role and responsibility necessary for their membership in society. This happens when fulfilling social responsibilities and continuing to belong to society are threatened. With their silence, the children maintain their relationship to the other players in the game. They demonstrate (Inkeles 1968) that they can respond to the paradigms of the social order and to the personal needs of other individuals with whom they have direct contact.

A further reason may be that parents lose their leadership role in relationship to their child when he or she becomes sick. They cannot protect the child from the hospital and the procedures linked to it, and they can no longer raise their child. They increasingly lose their authority and their ability to provide guidance. And in the end, leukemia "takes" their child from them. In a certain way, this development helps parents prepare for parting. Of course many parents try to protect their children from knowing because they believe the children will be unhappy or will give up too soon. And the children play along because they sense that otherwise they will frighten their parents even more.

The task of the doctors and nurses is to cure the patient or at least to see to it that the patient gets better. They did not learn how to talk with someone who is dying during their training, but they were taught how to detach from a patient in order to complete their tasks. Bluebond-Langner also wrote about the fact that doctors have not learned to deal with medical failure. She quoted a doctor who said that "death represents failure to a physician and it's hard for him to deal with it." Glaser and Strauss (1967) commented that many doctors choose particular specialties like radiology or microbiology in order to avoid this problem. Many nurses admit that they prefer to work on wards where they are seldom confronted with death and the patients recover. So reciprocal deception also helps doctors protect their own role as healer. As long as they can pretend that the children will get better at some point, they are doing their duty.

I discuss Bluebond-Langner's comments from 1978 so thoroughly here because they provide an excellent picture of the typical situation up to the 1980s. Children were "condemned to silence," as the psychologist Wolff described it. Bluebond-Langner's chapter is still worth reading today because there are still doctors who behave as she describes, and her comments allow us to understand the reasons why. In the countries behind the Iron Curtain, this approach was still the standard at the beginning of the 1990s.

In closing the chapter, Bluebond-Langner told of two of the children she studied who established the context of open awareness with their parents on their own initiative. These parents were different from all of the others in that they did not define their identity solely through their role as parents, and they worried less than other parents about what society thought and expected from them. With this as background, the conclusion the author reached at the end is impossible to understand. She emphasized repeatedly that the children "are aware," yet she argued for persisting in reciprocal deception and not moving on to the final stage of open awareness. In her opinion, this behavioral concept helps the individual maintain the social order. Breaking the rules means risking expulsion and abandonment—a fate that is, as she wrote, worse than death itself.

In her conclusion, we see once more the ambivalence we have also observed in the comments of others. She was not a doctor and was not part of the treatment team, so she adopted the role of observer. She did describe how anger overcame her at the death of a child. She believed that children keep to the rules their parents provide them and are able to deal successfully with these rules; she also believed it is more important for children to have their parents with them than to hear their prognosis. She never answered the reader's question of what we should actually communicate to children. She did construct a list of behaviors that allow us to assess the extent of the sick child's awareness:

- avoidance of deceased children's names and belongings
- lack of interest in conversation and play not related to the disease
- preoccupation with death and disease imagery in play, art, and literature
- engagement of selected individuals in conversations about factors that reveal or conceal
- anxiety about increased debilitation and about going home, but for different reasons than earlier in the disease process
- avoidance of talk about the future
- concern that things be done immediately (don't lose any time!)
- refusal to cooperate with relatively simple, painless procedures
- distancing from others through displays of anger or silence.

In my opinion, these behavior patterns are valid predominantly for children with whom no one talks (mutual pretense), and the picture is quite different when we talk openly with them, including about death and dying. Let's keep in mind, though, that Bluebond-Langner too was convinced that the children knew about their prognosis. Eighteen years later she published another book (1996) dealing with the influence of serious illness on children and their siblings and parents; it is comforting to know that she drew very different conclusions and in fact urged that the context be one of open awareness, the very approach she had expressly rejected in the book discussed here. In even later publications (2003, 2006), she left absolutely no doubt that open communication with sick children is the right way to support them and not abandon them in their distress. "Children's Views of Death," a contribution to a 2006 textbook on palliative care for children written with Amy DeCicco, should be recommended reading (Bluebond-Langner and DeCicco 2006).

In 1978, the same year Bluebond-Langner published her first book, Swiss child and adolescent psychiatrist Dieter Bürgin published his book *Das Kind, die lebensbedrohende Krankheit und der Tod* (The child, life-threatening illness, and death). He dealt extensively with the development of death concepts in children and in the process reported on the studies of healthy children by psychoanalysts and developmental psychologists discussed earlier in this book. He adopted Piaget's multistage model more or less without contradiction and devoted only a brief section to sick children. He referred almost exclusively to the reports by Raimbault, whose book was published in France in 1975. He quoted her observations that all children are aware that death threatens, but he made no further comment on this fact.

Bürgin did conclude at the end of the book that "a life-threatening illness leads to an acceleration of children's emotional development and probably of their cognitive development as well. Through the effects of the treatment this acceleration of maturity creates an enormous surplus burden for a child's ego." With regard to providing the children with information, he referred only to the Paris group (Bernard and Alby 1956; Alby and Alby 1971). In the end, his statements remain vague. This book also dealt with children who had leukemia, and oncologists in German-speaking countries certainly took note of it, but it did not change doctors' fundamental failure to consider children's attempts to deal with death. This was equally true of the analogous chapter in the *Handbuch der Kinderpsychotherapie* (Handbook of child psychotherapy) that appeared in 1981 (Hennigsen and Ullner 1981).

In 1983, an edited volume with the title *The Child and Death* was published in the United States. In one chapter, A. R. Zweig summarized the state of knowledge at the time: children often don't talk about death, they know nothing about their parents' attitude toward death, and yet by the age of eight they have developed a fear of death. The most important influences on the development of their concepts of death, in his opinion, are the parents' attitude toward the question and the way they talk about it with their child. All of the other articles in the book that deal with death concepts in any way didn't go beyond the views of developmental psychologists described earlier.

Psychiatrist Elisabeth Kübler-Ross published her book *On Children and Death* in the same year. She made a major contribution by moving death and dying into public consciousness. In most of her books she deals with adults, but this book is about sick children and their families. In the introduction, she wrote: "There are thousands of children who know death far beyond the knowledge adults have. Adults may listen to these children and shrug it off; they may think that children do not comprehend death; they may reject their ideas. But one day they may remember these teachings, even if it is only decades later when they face 'the ultimate enemy' themselves. Then they will discover that those little children were the wisest of teachers, and they, the novice pupils."

Kübler-Ross raised many important questions in the introduction and attempts to answer them. But in what follows, she did not proceed systematically, so it isn't easy to decipher her answers. In a letter to parents who had lost a child, she wrote about the knowledge children have that they often don't communicate to adults. She also emphasized that all children have knowledge (intuitive, not conscious) about the outcome of their illness. And since everyone, whether old or young, needs someone he or she can confide in, the children choose such a person; it is often another child. Bluebond-Langner wrote that the children often carry on brief conversations; adults would be amazed by what they say. She did idealize the situation when she asserted that God balances things out by making the children stronger in inner wisdom and intuitive knowledge as the little ones' bodies break down. Of course this was also intended as consolation for the parents to whom the letter is written. Kübler-Ross was also convinced that this is true, thus occupying the same metaphysical plane as Asperger, whose ideas about the "precociously mature" child were discussed in chapter 7 (Asperger 1969).

Kübler-Ross was also not particularly interested in concepts; she was convinced of the children's knowledge and supported her viewpoint with a few anecdotes. Developmental psychologists were probably not convinced, but presumably she had little interest in that. She wanted adults to take children seriously, so she didn't shrink from making some broad generalizations. Although I share her opinion about the knowledge seriously ill children possess and above all about the necessity for adults to take children seriously, this book cannot be viewed as a scientific work. Written more with the nonprofessional public in mind, it can help convince parents to talk about life and death with their children.

In 1984 a book that involved the participation of many authors was published in the United States under the title *Childhood and Death* (Wass and Corr 1984). Eugenia Waechter, who had written an article about what children know about death in 1971, wrote a chapter on the same topic for this book. She had already reported in her first article that young children know about their own death and can talk about it. Here she reported on a study of fifty-six sick children between the ages of four and ten. Almost all of the parents had gotten involved in a conversation with their children about diagnosis and death. They reported almost without exception that children over five knew a lot about their illness. And even four-year-olds gave clues that they knew about their prognosis.

Waechter also distanced herself from developmental concepts based on Piaget and reported her observations of the various age groups. Preschool children, whose concept of causality is not yet mature, often blame themselves for their illness. If their parents don't talk with them about it, this feeling can become more intense. The children feel their parents are rejecting them when they have to enter the hospital, and this makes the feeling that they are being punished even stronger. They often become more withdrawn. They are also frightened about being furious with their parents, on whom they are dependent. Waechter clarified how much sick toddlers need their parents in order to deal with their feelings. Children need constant assurance that their parents love them and that they will not be abandoned or rejected.

At this point, we need to investigate what this author had to say about toddlers' fear of death. Waechter believed that toddlers do not yet have a complete concept of death, but at four children are definitely able to understand that other living things have become nonexistent. Linked to their guilt feelings, the fear that they will be abandoned forever may develop in some children. Parents report that toddlers don't talk about death, but their anxieties become apparent in their behavior. Nightmares, behavioral changes, increased aggressiveness in play, worrying about the death of other children, and many other things point to the presence of fear. There are other children who simply don't allow themselves to think about nonexistence. They don't ask any questions and repress their feelings. This is the approach these children need until death is near. Regressing to a more childlike behavior allows them to be dependent on their parents; they need assurance from their parents that they will not be left alone with the unforeseeable.

In Waechter's opinion, schoolchildren between six and ten need reciprocal communication. They ask questions, and they are aware that they could die. The author referred to the article by John J. Spinetta and Lorrie J. Maloney (1975), who ten years earlier had studied the communicative behavior of children with cancer and how it was linked to their handling of the situation of being ill. Like these authors, Waechter thought that when parents and doctors opt for silence and avoidance, it can lead children to deny the situation and leave them with a feeling of being isolated and rejected. Open communication at the child's request can lead to family members supporting each other. Waechter did point out that Spinetta and Maloney thought that forced openness, especially if it comes too early, can be destructive and lead to serious problems with coping. Waechter didn't restrict herself to school-children's concepts of death and instead described her own observations. In the case of adolescents, her main interest was how people at that age deal with their imminent death.

In the same book, H. Wass discussed children's concepts of death at length. In her survey of the literature, she observed that many authors agreed with Piaget and his theory of cognitive development. She too was convinced that concepts of death develop in a well-ordered way, from incomprehension through limited understanding to complete understanding. There is little variation in the sequence of individual steps, assuming the children's environment remains constant. But children vary widely in their development, and they reach the stages Piaget defined at various ages. She believed, however, that it was a mistake to assume that cognitive development is strictly dependent on the age-related maturation of the child. No one develops in a social vacuum, and influences from the environment are significant, a fact that Piaget did not address. So it didn't contradict his theories when severely ill or dying children understand death much earlier and move through the various steps of cognitive development at very different ages than healthy children. Wass felt that her position is also validated by John Bowlby's work (1980).

In a later chapter of their book *Childhood and Death*, H. Wass and L. Cason looked at the fear of death from another perspective. One section deals with the influence of children's experience on fear and anxieties. In the meantime, psychoanalysts and psychologists are in agreement that childhood is an important time for the development of anxieties; both perceive the parents' role in early childhood as vital. It is Freud's opinion that the adult personality is formed exclusively during the first six years and that all dysfunctions in adults go back to this time. According to him, the first six years of life are full of unconscious anxieties such as castration anxiety. Freud believed that these neurotic problems are unavoidable and that children and their parents must solve them somehow.

One must ask, however, how parents are supposed to do this if they don't ever find out about these anxieties? This view of human development completely neglects the influence of environment. Wass and Cason cited A. W. Combs and associates (1976), who asserted that the development of self-conception begins at birth and becomes more sophisticated through the interaction between children and their environment. They believed that traumatic experiences such as birth, death, or the divorce of parents do have a certain influence on children's self-understanding but that this influence has been overstated. In their view, the daily interactions between children and their parents and others are much more important.

Wass and Cason clarified the impact of parents' behavior. If, for example, parents' love is tied to conditions, then children learn that they are valued under certain conditions but will be rejected under others. This kind of volatility can definitely be a fundamental cause of anxieties. Thus these authors too assumed that how parents and people in the child's environment behave will also have a definite influence on how concepts of death develop as well as a strong influence on the development of the child's self-esteem. Myra Bluebond-Langner (1978) had already determined that a child's "self-concept" plays a fundamental role in dealing with the fear of death. A child's experience in life is a crucial determining factor in his or her cognitive development. As I pointed out earlier, this does not mean a complete rejection of the developmental stages defined by Piaget.

In 1985 an American working group made up of Ruprecht Nitschke and his colleagues reported on their general concepts relating to the care of chronically ill children with a progressive disease course. In 1977 and 1982 they had described their experiences including children in the final stage of their illness in the process of deciding for or against an experimental therapy (1977). The 1985 study appeared in the most important German journal in pediatrics (Nitschke et al. 1985). The authors wrote that at the time of diagnosis, they told all children older than five that they have a cancer that will be fatal without treatment. The children (and parents) were assured that they will be truthfully informed about the course of the disease, even when the disease is progressing despite treatment and a cure seems impossible.

This course of action is based on four observations made repeatedly by the authors:

- The diagnosis cannot be concealed from the children.
- Children know that death is an irrevocable event.
- Children are able to grapple with their own death.
- Half-truths used by a doctor to explain the disease situation are unsatisfactory for the doctor and disturb the relationship between doctor and child.

Nitschke and his collaborators indicated that the first three points are convincingly documented in the literature (Bennholdt-Thomsen 1959; Vernick and Karon 1965; Reilly et al. 1983), but they also indicated that the fourth statement reflected their personal opinion, so the views of other doctors may differ. These authors spent little time considering concepts of death, since they too are convinced that children do have the pertinent knowledge.

In a paper published two years later, the same working group investigated the differences in death concepts between healthy children and children with cancer (Jay et al. 1987). The authors also wanted to find out whether having an earlier experience with death played a role for sick children, and whether there were illness-related factors that influenced their concept formation. They studied thirty-two sick children between three and sixteen years old and contrasted them with an equal group of healthy children of the same ages. The following subconcepts were investigated:

- Animism: everything that moves is alive.
- Anthropomorphism: the reason for human motivation, human characteristics, or human behavior lies in inanimate objects or the dead.
- Causality (justice): sin or guilt is the cause of death
- Causality (concrete): the biological cause is understood in principle. Death means the end of life.
- Causality (abstract): death occurs through the failure of bodily functions. Invisible things such as internal biology are the causes.
- Universality: all people must die.
- Personal death: I too can die.
- Irrevocability: the dead cannot come back to life.

The groups differed noticeably in their ideas about two subconcepts. For a third of the healthy children, the concept of punishment (punishment for sin or guilt) was present, while this was not true, surprisingly, for any of the children with cancer. It is even more surprising that almost all of the healthy children understood the subconcept of "personal death," while it was only demonstrable in a third of the children with cancer. The two groups did not differ with regard to the other subconcepts. In the cancer group (only investigated in that group), the development of some subconcepts was found to be clearly dependent on the number of people the child knew who had died. For the subconcepts "universality," "personal death," and "irrevocability," the difference was significant only for the children between three and six years of age and not for the older children. No other significant correlations were found.

The sick children in this study may not have demonstrated a concept of personal death because they were repressing it out of fear; in any case, that was the authors' interpretation. It is even more difficult to understand the difference between the groups with regard to the concept of punishment. Here, too, the authors asked themselves whether the sick children were frightened by the possibility of being punished for a sin or for wrongdoing. In my own experience, children often consider this when they are looking for a reason for their illness. The other explanation the authors discussed is that the sick children probably have already received detailed explanations for the cause of the disease, so that this concept is no longer available to them, in contrast to the healthy children. The recognition that experience plays an important part for young children confirms the earlier findings of B. Kane (1979) and Thomas P. Reilly and collaborators (1983); concepts that can be directly experienced or observed are more easily influenced by experience than concepts that are dependent on cognitive abilities. The author Susan M. Jay did recommend a certain amount of skepticism, since the number of children in the individual groups was quite small. Nevertheless, the article confirms that children between three and six can develop concepts of death, a fact that is important for the care of sick children.

Another article from the same time compared healthy and sick children (Clunies-Ross and Lansdown 1988). This working group had published a study of 195 healthy children from 1985 that showed that young children— some only four or five years old—are able to develop a realistic concept of death (Lansdown and Benjamin 1985). In the later study, they looked at twenty-one children with leukemia using the same method: the children were questioned after they were told a story about a woman who had died. Clunies-Ross and Lansdown discovered that the conceptual development of the sick children did not differ in any fundamental way from that of the healthy children. It is true that the younger sick children did seem to have a better understanding of some of the subconcepts than the healthy children did. The authors tried to find out what kind of understanding the sick children had of the reason for their illness. They were amazed to find that none of the children gave the correct explanation. In closing, Clunies-Ross and Lansdown pointed out that the findings for children under eight were quite variable, and they warned against generalizing them for application in the hospital.

In the interest of completeness, I discuss two German dissertations published in 1988 and 1994. The first is by educator and psychologist H. Iskenius-Emmler (1988). By describing the state of scientific debate at that time, she gave the reader a good overview, particularly with regard to children and grief. She discussed the literature of developmental psychology and psychoanalysis thoroughly and concluded that young children too can carry out grief work with the appropriate cognitive and emotional support and cope with a loss in that way. In her opinion, difficulties that arise as children work through grief result much more often from adults' behavior than from the immaturity of the child's ego. This attitude is probably based in large part on her intensive critical examination of articles published ten years earlier by psychologist G. Wolff (1978), who had a great deal of experience with children with cancer and was convinced that they knew much more than was commonly maintained at the time.

The second dissertation is by the sociologist G. Ramachers (1994). He addressed the issue of contradictions in the literature, reporting them primarily based on the surveys done by M. W. Speece and S. B. Brent (1984). He concluded that our view of the development of ideas about death is incomplete. With regard to the development of cognitive understanding of the primary components (subconcepts) of the death concept, by and large the findings seem to be consistent. But in the opinion of Ramachers, their emotional meaning is still open to interpretation. Here he cited a problem with our understanding that other authors had already expressed.

The same problem is identified in another article that investigates what children with cancer see and feel (Claflin and Barbarin 1991). After studying the literature, the authors concluded that it is too early to make a definitive statement about the limits of children's cognitive abilities and their ability to regulate emotional disturbances. They too emphasized how important experience is—here, experience with cancer—for the development of death concepts. They closed by saying that "methods currently used to study cognitive coping strategies of young children (including our own) fail to uncover fully the range of cognitions they employ."

Another study on this topic from the perspective of developmental psychology was published in 1990 (Cotton and Range 1990). The authors studied forty-two children between the ages of six and twelve. The subjects were selected; all were white children from a Bible study class. Two-thirds of the children reported experiences with death in their close proximity. An analysis of the data showed that the strongest predictive factors for the existence of death concepts were the extent of cognitive development (positive correlation) and earlier experience with death (negative correlation). The second finding contradicted the results of Reilly and his collaborators (1983), who viewed experience as a catalytic factor that accelerated the developmental process. The authors speculated that the children's religious background might explain the different results. The religious belief in life after death might have led to the children misunderstanding the cause of death and its inevitability. Apart from that, the authors found that understanding of death was dependent much more on the children's cognitive development than on their age. In the case of these healthy children, hopelessness was not correlated with the overall development of concepts of death. These authors too were cautious about the significance of their data because of the small number of cases.

In the years that followed, studies concentrated on the question of whether we should tell children they are dying and, if so, what we should tell them. In the oncology literature, it is increasingly assumed that this is the critical question. This topic is covered in chapter 10, and we will see that even today, there is still no unanimous opinion on this issue.

The final publication I would like to discuss here is the book *Never Too Young to Know—Death in Children's Lives* by Phyllis R. Silvermann, which was published in the United States in 2000. She writes that toddlers between one and a half and three years of age do not yet have a concept of death, but they are able to accept the loss that is connected to death as continuous. She too adheres to the levels of understanding Piaget described but emphasizes that adults can help children go through the levels more quickly by providing adequate information. In her opinion, a six-year-old can understand death's inevitability, its finality, and the essential aspects of the biological processes connected to it.

Conclusion

In chapter 8, on the death concepts of healthy children, research by psychoanalysts and developmental psychologists since the beginning of the twentieth century was reviewed in detail. There have been few new findings in this area since the 1980s. Since that time, interest has focused increasingly on children who are sick or dying, and the authors are more often pediatricians, particularly pediatric oncologists, and pediatric nurses. Well into the 1970s, based on developmental concepts that were primarily psychoanalytic, it was easy for pediatricians to deny that children had any understanding of death and dying. Their own fear of this topic, at a time when it was also a taboo topic for society in general, made it hard for them to accept that children too think about their own death. In the first half of the twentieth century, there was the additional reality that most severely ill children, such as children who had cancer, died quickly. For that reason it was possible to claim that there was little time to talk with children about death. In my opinion, this is not entirely accurate, since there were other chronic illnesses at that time, such as tuberculosis or osteomyelitis, that were often fatal because there were no medications for treating them. And often the children and adolescents died only after a lingering illness that lasted for months or even years, so there would have been plenty of time to talk with them.

It was more likely the subject of death and dying in connection with children that so alarmed pediatricians and society as a whole; it was not just the doctors who were helpless when confronted by this kind of situation. The belief that children had faulty concepts of death or lacked them entirely served as a good excuse for not talking with them about the topic.

In this chapter, I have traced the scientific development chronologically. At the beginning of the second half of the twentieth century, researchers hesitantly began to address the question of whether the development of a death concept might proceed differently in sick children than in healthy ones. Developmental psychologists alluded to the question often, and there was occasional cautious speculation that there might be differences in the developmental process between healthy and sick children. In the 1950s two studies of children with cancer appeared, showing for the first time that sick children clearly knew more than people had previously thought (Bernard and Alby 1956; Bennholdt-Thomson 1959). Bennholdt-Thomson reported the observations made by his collaborators almost with amazement and at least came to the conclusion that more research should be done. Bernard and Alby, on the other hand, arrived at an unexpected conclusion. They found that children notice and understand more of hospital routine than had previously been thought. But their conclusion was that everything possible should be done to prevent them from acquiring this knowledge.

As a result, German and Swiss authors cited these statements again and again, emphasizing that children lack concepts of death and also don't want to know anything about it. Results from studies of healthy children were cited repeatedly as evidence for the correctness of this way of thinking. Even the two psychotherapists Wunnerlich (1972) and Raimbault (1977) remained trapped in the standard beliefs of their guild, although they had done an excellent job of portraying the attitudes of seriously ill and dying children in many case studies. They wanted above all to avoid the final and decisive step—talking with the children about the eventuality of death or about the fact that the children might die. From today's point of view, the children's behavior virtually demanded openness. These two authors were less interested in describing the development of concepts of death than in describing the behaviors and ideas of the children they had observed.

In the second half of the twentieth century, these concepts played a smaller role for other authors as well; instead, they reported their observations of children's behavior. Increasingly, doctors actively involved in caring for sick children are the source of publications rather than developmental psychologists or psychoanalysts. And the question of whether and how we should talk with children is addressed more often. I have devoted so much attention to the literature because I believe that open communication with children about death and dying is only possible and meaningful if they have or at least can develop definite concepts for what might or, in some cases, definitely will face them: death. Therefore, the two chapters on the development of death concepts by healthy and sick children differ in clear ways.

In the literature of the last thirty years it has become much clearer that the developmental stages posited by Piaget are not fundamentally incorrect and reflect what actually happens with healthy children relatively well. He himself pointed to children's individuality in this regard. Both psychoanalysis and Piaget put too little weight on children's experience, which may not change the sequence but can substantially accelerate the timing. If someone close to them dies, even very young children can experience the irrevocability of death. Beginning with the fourth year of life at the latest, children can develop a concept of death based on the influence of their own experience that permits them to cope with this threatening event. Parents play an essential role. If they answer their children's questions about death willingly and openly from the start and don't shroud the issue in secrecy, it is much easier for the children to develop appropriate ideas. Young children are more successful at dealing with concepts they can understand on the basis of their experience, while abstract topics remain inaccessible to them for a longer time.

Let us keep one thing in mind: everything points to the fact that even young children are able to develop both their own concept of death and a fear of death. These concepts depend more on experience than on age and therefore do not necessarily conform to adults' concepts. But they suffice for understanding a life-threatening disease and for working through the problems connected to it. Today it is no longer acceptable to cite children's lack of knowledge as justification for inadequate communication or no communication at all. As a result we are turning away from the protective silence we clung to during the first seven decades of the last century and turning toward communication that is open and informative—in other words, toward a concept of open truth.

CHAPTER TEN

Should We Tell Sick Children the Truth?

The question of whether we should be truthful with severely ill children about the state of their health gained in importance during the second half of the twentieth century. Until that time, the established medical doctrine was to leave severely ill and dying patients in the dark and to lie to them. I dealt with this topic at some length in chapter 9. In his book *The Silent World of Doctor and Patient,* Jay Katz (1984, 2002) covered this issue thoroughly. Since Hippocrates, doctors have withheld the truth from their patients, vehemently defended the practice, and found moral arguments to support their actions. We saw earlier how at the beginning of the nineteenth century, the famous physician Christoph Wilhelm Hufeland stated, "He who names death, brings death." The established principle was to talk only about positive things—or say nothing at all.

An Ongoing Controversy

In 1927, Dr. J. Collins published an article with the title "Should Doctors Tell the Truth?" in a popular magazine in the United States. He concluded:

The longer I practice medicine the more I am convinced that every physician should cultivate lying as a fine art. But there are many varieties of lying. Some are most prejudicial to the physician's usefulness. Such are: pretending to recognize the disease and understand its nature when one is really ignorant; asserting that one has effected the cure which nature has accomplished, or claiming that one can effect cure of a disease which is universally held to be beyond the power of nature or medical skill. . . . There are other lies, however, which contribute enormously to the success of the physician's mission of mercy and salvation.

This approach was ultimately the basis for doctors' paternalistic behavior over the centuries. A great many arguments were marshaled in support. The most important was surely that a doctor should never take away hope. In a critical article published in 1996 and titled "Should We Always Tell Children the Truth?" the American pediatrician John D. Lantos lists four reasons that doctors' behavior has changed and has become more communicative in the course of recent decades:

1. *Informed consent.* Doctors know a lot more about diseases today. Often they recognize a problem through laboratory tests or an X-ray (in the course of a medical checkup or during a screening, for example) before the patient even realizes he or she is sick, and then he or she must be informed. So an era of informed consent has developed. Patients are supposed to decide themselves what should be done. And to do this, they need information. Thus medicine is reacting less and less to medical crises and is instead becoming a health-related consumer product, much like a smoke detector or an airbag.

2. *High toxicity of therapies.* Many surgical measures and even nonsurgical measures make patients sick who were actually feeling fine. A good example is chemotherapy for leukemia in children, which causes them a lot of suffering in the interest of regaining their health. Patients must be informed about this in advance.

3. *Multiple therapy options.* In many cases, there are several therapy options. That means that doctor and patient have to decide on one of the possibilities, and to do this they have to exchange information.

4. *A change in basic attitude.* Both doctor and patient increasingly view medicine as an undertaking in which progress is perpetual and unrelenting. This progress, however, is only possible due to research, which leads to new agreements between doctor and patient and to a

detailed disclosure of the facts. After major difficulties early on, ethical guidelines for research on humans that were intended to protect patients, such as the Declaration of Helsinki, were developed. The prerequisite is clear and unambiguous information for the patient. I don't want to gloss over the fact that the development of the declaration was a consequence of experiments on humans by National Socialist doctors in Germany.

There are certainly many justifiable reasons for the introduction of informed consent. But the problems it can pose if doctors use it only to protect themselves instead of first and foremost to enlighten and inform the patient have already been described in the discussion of paternalism and autonomy in chapter 6. Lantos gets to the heart of the matter when he writes that articles about informed consent should fall under the rubric of risk management, not patient autonomy. And in fact, legal arguments are not always congruent with ethical principles. Of course the principle behind informed consent is not fundamentally wrong. But we do have to ask ourselves whether many doctors act in accordance with it for their own personal advantage and thus not in the patient's best interest. This same development has also taken place in pediatrics.

This has been a brief background for what follows, when we look at whether these changes in adult medicine have also had consequences for handling the truth with sick children and adolescents, and if it has, what the results have been. I first trace this development and then close with a recommendation that can and must serve as a basis for hospital practice. One thing needs to be said in advance, and for this purpose I quote Lantos, who writes,

> Following the ancient moral tradition, doctors learned to withhold potentially stressful information, to conceal bleak diagnoses, and not to discuss the risks of treatments or procedures. In doing so, doctors were following the moral maxim of either saying nice things or else saying nothing at all. In light of this history, recent moral sentiment that patients ought to be told the truth—the whole truth—no matter how horrible it might be or how ill prepared they might be to hear it represents one of those mysterious changes in morality that occur from time to time, whereby something that once was thought morally intolerable rather suddenly comes to be thought of as morally obligatory.

Lantos exaggerates the situation, and we could get the impression that the modern form of information provision is fundamentally bad. You don't provide moral justification for the principle of providing information by expressing it in a harsh and unsparing way, with the object of conveying all available information to the patient. Instead, doctors today need to develop the ability to proceed in the patient's interest, and they must understand that protecting themselves cannot be the objective.

In the course of reviewing various publications in the chapter on the death concepts of sick children, I repeatedly discussed what the authors had to say about informing children about their illness and its consequences. From the way they proceeded, in other words how prepared they were to talk openly with children about their illness, we can infer how much confidence they had in the children. We can also tell whether they assumed that most children have some knowledge about death and made this assumption the basis of their work. I tried to make it clear that the majority of authors had and still have great difficulty with openly informing sick children.

In this chapter, the developmental process in pediatric and adolescent medicine will be summarized once again; its endpoint is the recognition of the young person as a being who thinks and acts independently and whose needs the doctor must understand in order to be correspondingly helpful and supportive for those who are seriously ill. So I will refer once more to studies mentioned in earlier chapters, this time with respect to their positions on providing information. If we want to learn how to behave when dealing with dying children, we need to understand how children think. It is equally necessary to understand why so many doctors had and still have difficulty dealing openly with children and communicating with them. There is no doubt that children and adolescents open up only to people who approach them openly.

The sick children who are the subjects of this chapter almost all have cancer. Pediatricians who treat children with cancer are obviously confronted with dying children most often, although some of the articles discussed earlier were by psychologists, specialists in therapeutic education, social workers, and pediatric nurses. Open communication plays an especially important role for these children. It is clear that the way doctors' behavior developed was significantly influenced by advances in oncology since the Second World War. The following brief summary of these advances is provided in the interest of better understanding.

Until 1950 there were no prospects for a cure for children with acute leukemia, and therefore they often died quickly. In 1948 the Boston pathologist

Sydney Farber was able to demonstrate that a temporary remission of leukemia in these children was achieved with the injection of the folic acid antagonist aminopterin, although the children were not cured. Aminopterin was soon replaced by the analogue amethopterin (methotrexate), which is still one of the standard medications for treating the most common form of childhood leukemia. Later, other medications were discovered that, when administered in succession, led to a lengthening of the period of remission during which the leukemia was not detectable, and some children survived for two or even three years. But a treatment-resistant relapse always occurred at some point, and the children died as a result. In Memphis during the second half of the 1960s, Donald Pinkel did several sequential studies whose results were first published in 1971. He demonstrated that combination therapy together with prophylactic cranial irradiation could lead to a long-term cure in a small percentage of children. And in the early 1970s in Berlin, Hansjörg Riehm and his collaborators demonstrated the correctness of his hypothesis that all medications that have been shown to be effective when administered individually must be administered at the beginning of therapy to prevent the leukemic cells from developing a resistance to any one of them. By the mid-1970s it became clear that with this treatment half of the children could survive; today it is more than two-thirds. By now this is also true for solid malignant tumors, which also can often be cured.

One point is particularly important in the context of this chapter. Originally all children with cancer died. In the period following the first successful cancer therapy, sick children began to survive for longer periods. Later, more and more often, they were cured. As a result, these children had more time to deal with their illness and everything connected with it. In the long term, the caregivers could not avoid paying more attention to these children and their thinking. In this chapter we will carefully retrace this process.

I mentioned earlier that in 1959 the German pediatrician Bernhard de Rudder made the general observation that many children die before "their soul knows a longing for death." With this formulation he stands in the shadow of Freud, who at the beginning of the twentieth century had denied that children had any understanding of death. The first article on the psychological aspects of caring for children with cancer was published in 1955 in the United States (Richmond and Waisman 1955). In it, the authors questioned the level of knowledge of children and adolescents. They reported that the young patients almost never ask questions, although adults often do.

Perhaps, they speculated, this behavior isn't a signal that they don't want to know; it may be a defense mechanism against the fear of death. These authors did not develop clear ideas of how we should deal with children and adolescents; instead, they addressed the problems of parents and caregivers much more intensively. They didn't even entertain the question of whether we should speak openly with children.

The following year, a study by a working group in Paris was published (Bernard and Alby 1956) in which the authors portrayed in detail how children as young as three are able to express their fear of death. They described fairly precisely how severely ill children are able to arrive at their insights and that all dying children are familiar with the threat of death—even at the age of four or five. But Bernard and Alby still didn't conclude that we should talk with children about their diagnosis, dying, and death. Instead they described carefully all the things adults have to keep in mind in order to hide these dire facts. They pointed out that terminally ill adults are also not informed truthfully.

In his book *Kind, Krankheit und Tod* (The child, illness, and death), published in 1957, child psychiatrist Erich Stern reported at length about the experiences of children who had come in contact with death in their environment and at age four were already afraid of it. He did not discuss how to deal with dying children in his book; the reason may be that he had only provided psychotherapy to children who were suffering from the effects of experiences with death.

In 1959 Carl-Gottlieb Bennholdt-Thomsen, professor of pediatric medicine in Cologne, published his study about death and dying in children, in which he reported on individual children who had died. As far as I know, he was the first pediatrician to address specifically this topic in a German medical journal, although the observations were not his own but those of his collaborators. He pointed out that these issues were not addressed in any pediatric textbook, even though no pediatrician is spared the experience of children dying. He asked what the field of pediatrics actually knows about what goes on inside a dying child and noted that there are only two monographs by psychologists on this topic (Illig and Bates-Ames 1955; Stern 1957). He quoted the Dutch philosopher Baruch Spinoza, who said that "a free man thinks of death least of all things; and his wisdom is a meditation not of death but of life."

Bennholdt-Thomsen pondered whether Spinoza's statement is correct or whether he should instead endorse the view of psychologist and educational theorist Gerhard Pfahler, who said, "Human beings, even when they are adult and mature, would not be living human beings if the word death lost all its uncanny quality and its horror." He also wanted to find out how children confront anxiety and fear of death and dying and how they behave when anxiety and fear become unavoidable reality.

With an approach based on actual case histories (he used the clinical term *casuistics*), he hoped to find answers to these questions. He incorporated clinical observations by doctors and nurses of children's statements shortly before their death and of statements by sick children who recovered. The children in the first group said clearly that they knew death was approaching. The children in the second group also expressed their fear of death, but they lacked, as Bennholdt-Thomsen observed, the unmistakable feeling of the nearness of death. The children in the first group were not wrong in their awareness that death would come soon. Bennholdt-Thomsen gave a great deal of thought to the reports; this is apparent in his article, which he closed with a reflective passage. He did not try to evade the fact that children know about death and talk about it. Instead, he challenged the reader to reflect on it. But it still didn't occur to him to talk with the children; instead, he reported how they tried to calm a child who "knew" about his death by leaving behind a falsified medical record.

In 1960, two American pediatricians, one of whom, Knudson, was also a cancer geneticist, published two articles about their approach to involving parents in the care of their terminally ill children in the hospital (Knudson and Natterson 1960) and about the fear of death of the children and their mothers (Natterson and Knudson 1960). They too reported that children clearly confront death early and are able to develop a fear of death when they hear that another child has died. They described three patterns of behavioral changes in reaction to changes in their environment. Up to the age of five, the children react most strongly to separations; the reactions to procedures were strongest in five- to ten-year-olds; and children who were even older developed the most pronounced fear of death. But they didn't say a word about any conclusions they might have drawn from their observations—for example, the need for more openness in interacting with these children.

German-speaking pediatricians who wrote about the care of children with leukemia at the time also failed to encourage openness or didn't even mention the issue (Oehme et al. 1958; Hertl 1961; Hitzig 1965). The American social worker James Morrissey (1963) described children's anxieties in great detail and concluded that a third are definitely conscious of the seriousness of the situation. Supporting these children is difficult, in his opinion. He saw it as essentially a task in the realm of social work but didn't elaborate on how it should be done.

Then, in 1965, the article by social worker Joel Vernick and pediatrician Myron Karon with the provocative title "Who's Afraid of Death on a Leukemia Ward?" was published; I discussed it at length in chapter 10 in the section on the death concepts of sick children. These authors argued strongly for openness, since all children know what is happening to them. They determined that parents are unable to hide their worries from the children no matter how hard they try. Children quickly sense that the people they trust are now trying to hide something from them, as if they were saying, "Please don't ask me about this; it's too awful." All fifty-one of the children in the study accepted the disclosure of their terminal diagnosis without any defensive reaction and often with relief, which convinced Vernick and Karon that their approach had been the right one. The team was able to relinquish the traditional approach of "protection through concealment" and as a result was able to help the children cope with their fears. In closing, they emphasized that everyone on a leukemia ward is troubled by fear, and eliminating it is a problem everyone shares.

This article's conclusions are unambiguous and don't allow for any qualifications, so we can only be surprised that something like it could have been written more than forty years ago. The authors' intensive discussions with their collaborators probably contributed a great deal to their absolute certainty that their actions in the children's interest were right. They were ahead of their time, and we have to ask how that happened. Ten years later, when I began providing information to children because I was becoming increasingly certain it was the right approach, I had not yet read the study. At the time, we were not able to find interesting publications simply by typing certain keywords into a computer search engine. I discovered the article many years later, but I can remember as if it were yesterday how happy I was to find my concept confirmed. At that time, openness in dealing with severely ill children had not yet made its appearance in German hospitals and probably not in American hospitals either.

Judging from the editorial in the next volume of the same American journal, it is clear that not everyone agreed with Vernick and Karon's work (Agranoff and Mauer 1965). Agranoff and Mauer, both pediatricians interested in the treatment of children and adolescents with cancer, were concerned about the effects of openness on the children's relationship with their parents, siblings, or other relatives as well as with playmates and classmates. They acknowledged that the situation in a specialized hospital, such as the one where the group connected to Vernick and Karon worked, might be different than in their hospital, where children with leukemia were not on a separate ward. They thought it was probably more difficult to hide the truth from children in a hospital where all children with leukemia are together on a single ward. They believed there was far too little information available on which to base behavior toward children with leukemia, and therefore much more observation was needed. So competent authorities called the conclusions reached by the social worker Vernick and the pediatrician Karon into question. This must have conveyed to the pediatricians of the time that they didn't need to follow this example, and for a long time most doctors did not do so. And so nothing fundamental changed.

The two authors commented on this editorial in a letter (Vernick and Karon 1965). They explained that it was the very fears and anxieties mentioned in the editorial that had kept children from significant information in the past. They also did not believe there is a difference between children treated in a special pediatric leukemia hospital and those treated on wards with other children who don't have cancer. They emphasized once again that all children over five know how serious their illness is. They were convinced that the children's ostensible lack of interest described by other authors (Richmond and Waisman 1955) simply reflected the children's recognition that adults are not willing to discuss their serious problems with them. In the opinion of the two advocates of open dialogue, the "aftereffects of openness" feared by critics actually provide both the child and his environment with the basis for a constructive examination. The authors closed their letter by stating that they were concerned about children in general hospitals because they may have absolutely no one with whom they can discuss their problems. In addition, in this situation there are no other children with the same illness with whom they can communicate. This statement shows how far ahead of their time Vernick and Karon were in both their approach and their insights.

Two years later the second article by the Paris working group appeared that dealt with the psychological aspects of treating leukemia in children and young adults in a specialized treatment center (Alby et al. 1967). The authors discussed at length whether patients should be informed of their diagnosis. They quoted internal medicine cancer specialist Charles Mathé, who later became very well known, and his collaborators in Paris; all were strictly against informing the patient, and their explanation ran as follows: "In our country, patients who know that they have leukemia live with moral and physical discomfort." Alby and his group reported that this reason for not informing patients reflected the general attitude in French medical practice. They themselves, obviously not sure that this categorical position was always the right one, preferred to decide on a case-by-case basis. The discussion in this case refers only to severely ill adults; with regard to children, the authors referred to the earlier study done at their hospital (Bernard and Alby 1956).

The article "Children and Death" by London pediatrician Simon Yudkin appeared in the respected journal *Lancet* in the same year (1967). He was among the authors who ascribed a certain level of knowledge about death even to young children. Although some terminally ill children are afraid they may die, others are only alarmed by the behavior of their parents, who know about the approaching death of their child. In his summary, he wrote that these children should have the opportunity of talking about their situation. Admittedly, he had no answer to the question of whether older children should be told that they are going to die.

This article is worthwhile because it is written by an empathetic pediatrician who has thought a lot about the problems of dying children. He included himself when he reported on the incompetence of doctors that was frequently in evidence. In his view, the biggest failing of his own team is that they seldom got to know the dying children and their families well enough to respond with sufficient empathy to the children's needs. Since he addressed almost all aspects connected to the death of children in this article, we have to ask why it had so little influence on doctors' behavior. Perhaps the answer is that it reflected—albeit in a sympathetic and honest way—the helplessness of this particular pediatrician. The article also demonstrates well what mental hurdles the individual doctor had to overcome in order to speak with children openly and without constraints. Yudkin did not yet dare take the final step of telling children honestly that they were going to die.

In the same year, American pediatrician Morris Green published an article entitled "Care of the Dying Child" in which he referred to his work with Albert J. Solnit (Solnit and Green 1959; Solnit 1965). The article is the manuscript of a lecture he had given at a conference of American pediatricians. His impassioned plea for honesty and dependability with children is especially remarkable, and I support it without hesitation. He was convinced that children know when their illness is life-threatening due to circumstances such as daily medications, blood transfusions, or frequent stays in the hospital. He wrote that a child can forgive a doctor for almost anything but dishonesty. And finally, he argued for an honest answer when children ask whether they are going to die. He emphasized that we can answer yes only if we have discussed it with parents, since they might want to answer such a question themselves or prefer that it not be answered at all. This constraint is still valid today, and that is why an important task for the pediatrician is to convince parents that being open and truthful with dying children is the right approach. A certain tentativeness is apparent when he emphasized in closing that we need to study not only the death concepts of sick children but the method and contents of communication with them as well.

In a study that was similar in approach but reached different conclusions, American authors reported two years later on interviews with twenty-three parents of children who died of leukemia (Binger et al. 1969). I have discussed the article elsewhere, but I quote from it again here.

> It is a grave error to think that a child over four or five year of age who is dying of a terminal illness does not realize its seriousness and probable fatality. Repeatedly experience has shown us otherwise.
>
> We have seen the pathetic consequences of the loneliness of a fatally ill child who has no one with whom he may talk over his serious concerns because his parents are frequently trying to shield him from the diagnosis. His siblings or contemporaries also almost never act as a sounding board for release of his tensions. Whereas dying adults can express some of their feelings to their spouses, to mature and respected friends, to the clergy or to doctors, the dying child may have to deal alone with his fears, concerns and apprehensions and also cope with his own inner scheme of fantasies and "white lies" developed by his parents so that meaningful communication between the child and adults is prevented. . . . The question is not whether to talk about the diagnosis and prognosis (the child usually senses it), but rather how to let the child know that his concerns are shared and understood and that there is willingness to talk about them with him. Reassuring him that everything humanly possible will be done, that each discomfort that can be alleviated will be, and that all are ready to help in every possible way will allay many apprehensions.

Hope rests not only on life or death. Recognizing with the child what he already knows (that he has a fatal illness) opens up communication without which hope cannot be conveyed. Though he knows the worst can happen, hope can yet be imparted. He knows that lies will not be told to him, that he will not be deserted physically or emotionally. And that he can voice aloud his feelings of sadness, fear, helplessness, loss or anxiety.

In another book (Niethammer 2010), I discussed the question of how we can implement what has been said. But I would like to emphasize at this point that the cited authors recognized the need for open communication early and described the reasons clearly. By the end of the 1960s at the latest, everything should have been clear to everyone. Subsequently, we could see, however, that it was not yet possible to close the discussion, and even today it has not come to an end.

At the same time (1968), the well-known American pediatric oncologist Audrey Evans published an article in the *New England Journal of Medicine* with the title "If a Child Must Die." She argued that we should not tell a child his diagnosis; for example, we should characterize leukemia as severe anemia, which we can easily treat. A large part of the article deals with the dying child. She wrote that children seldom ask directly whether they are going to die; only teenagers would occasionally express their fear of death. Evans wrote that as a doctor, she would confirm the seriousness of the illness and the fact that she could understand the fear. However, she would tell the young person that she did not know when anyone is going to die. In addition, she would remind him or her that in the past she had always been able to improve his or her situation and that she had known children who were equally sick and who had returned to health. In closing, Evans pointed out that the current trend is to be more open with children.

The article by Vernick and Karon (1965), which expressed a different opinion from hers, is cited in Evans's bibliography but not discussed. This makes it clear that Evans was not at all in agreement with the concept of openness. She based her different approach on work in pediatric oncology in Boston, where Sidney Farber practiced according to the concept of comprehensive care for the child and his family, but this concept did not include the idea of dealing honestly with patients. This is perhaps not surprising, considering that the famous pathologist Farber was sixty-four at this point and had been shaped by a very different tradition.

The American pediatric surgeon C. Everett Koop (1969) felt certain that children know a great deal but want to protect their parents by not talking about it with them. He had talked openly with some children who were terminally ill and reported that he had experienced no problems in doing so. But he never reached the point of making a general recommendation. This was also true for German pediatrician P. Sachtleben (1970), who had experienced the practice of openness with children with cancer in the United States. He wrote about it and recommended it but without going into how he himself had handled it. At the opposite end of the scale, German pediatrician Karl-Heinz Schäfer (1972) strongly advised against speaking openly with children. I knew him quite well, and he was a role model in pediatrics for us younger doctors. But he was a typical representative of pediatrics as it was practiced at the time. He also was firmly of the opinion that children really don't want to know anything about death and that we should therefore not talk with them about it. In general they are not in a position to process truth in a rational way. For this reason, the doctor should not try to break through a child's naiveté by force, even in a crisis situation. Of course a forceful breakthrough would not be the preferred method. Schäfer's own adult fears may have colored the way he expressed himself.

I will mention an experience Schäfer described in his article because I find it so characteristic of that time. The story saddened me the first time I read it, and it still has the same effect today. Schäfer had presented his ideas about how to interact with dying children at a gathering of Protestant theologians. One of the listeners reported after the lecture that Martin Luther had fully informed his own ten-year-old daughter in a similar situation and that the child had died comforted and full of faith in God. Schäfer expressed doubt as to whether comparisons across centuries could really be made. Luther's time, milieu, and power of persuasion could not be generalized. As fate would have it, a few years later this theologian's grandson became ill with an incurable tumor at the same age. At the explicit request of the family, including the grandfather, the child died uninformed. It is regrettable that the grandfather adopted the pediatrician Schäfer as his role model and not Luther. Although Schäfer did not write anything about this child and his death, we have to assume that, like many children at the time, he died alone. This approach was not helpful to these children. The article by Vernick and Karon had obviously still not arrived in Germany seven years after its publication in the United States. But even in the United States, as I mentioned before, it did not go undisputed.

In 1970 the short but valuable book by psychiatrist William M. Easson, *The Dying Child: The Management of the Child or Adolescent Who Is Dying,* was published in the United States. The author began with a general chapter about concepts of death in which he stated that even children under five can develop an understanding of death: "From about five years of age and most certainly by seven years, the child who is dying knows that he is about to lose the warm and loving relationships he has."

He then gave a good description of how dying children learn from the reactions of those around them what approach to dying is preferred and to what extent they can reveal their fears and sufferings without frightening their parents too much. In two following chapters he discussed dying schoolchildren and adolescents, and he made clear in an impressive way how we should interact with these two age groups. He clearly had no doubt that honesty is the only correct approach when a child is dying. He wrote, "At this age, the grade school child has the emotional ability to face the prospect of dying and to reach out to his parents and to his family for comfort and understanding. . . . The grade school child knows that death means a final separation from his life. He appreciates now what he will miss when he dies, and he must mourn this loss as he leaves. He is liable to be sad and bitter because he does not want to go. He is lonely because he is traveling this journey alone. . . . The grade school child can always use the support and the understanding of those whom he trusts."

In the chapter about dying adolescents, Easson emphasized that everything can be much more difficult at this time of life because adolescents may be too proud and bitter to accept consolation in any form: "Defiant in the face of death, desperately proud and often painfully lonely, the younger adolescent may insist on going through death, fiercely independent to the end." Easson left no doubt that honesty is called for, but precisely at this age the patient may prefer to deny the truth, and we should not refuse him or her that option; the adolescent will make it clear through his questions how he wants it to be.

Easson's book is notable because it was written by a psychiatrist still firmly in the tradition of developmental psychology but who went far beyond the description of concepts and got intensively involved with dying children and adolescents. For him there was no longer any question whether we should give children honest answers. And at least in the case of adolescents, he saw the necessity of involving them in decisions about therapy. In several works that appeared at about the same time—books by Annemarie Wunnerlich and Ginette Raimbault, which I discuss next, and works by specialist in therapeutic education Emma Plank—we see ambivalence. This is not at all in evidence in Easson's work; he was sure where he stood.

The question of how children die was a central issue in Europe during the 1970s. I have already pointed to two books by psychotherapists who studied dying children extensively. Swiss psychologist Annemarie Wunnerlich (1972) investigated what children thought and knew in detail but shied away from the final step: openness. This shows the great ambivalence in her feelings. Despite all her experience, she could not bring herself to make a general recommendation for a truthful exchange of ideas with dying children. This is also true of Emma Plank (1973, 1979), an American specialist in therapeutic education whose ambivalence is strikingly clear. In chapter 9, I quoted Plank and described her inner conflict between demanding honesty and taking the decisive step toward complete openness. She is similar to Wunnerlich in this respect, because she portrayed the context absolutely correctly, only to shy away from the final and necessary conclusion.

French psychotherapist Ginette Raimbault (1977) related stories about severely ill and dying children effectively in her book *L'enfant et la mort. Des enfants malades parlent de la mort: problèmes de la clinique du deuil* (The child and death. Sick children talk about death: problems in grief therapy). In her mind, there was no doubt that children know a lot and that we must talk with them. She called for honesty without beating around the bush, and she sharply rebuffed her psychoanalytic predecessors and their concepts.

It is unfortunate that Raimbault didn't describe her own procedures in the individual stories. I can still remember well that I was constantly frustrated as I read this book because her description of the children's difficulties alone was not enough. I would have liked to find out how she had proceeded in each case and how she had communicated with the affected child and, possibly, was able to help and support him or her in his distress. Nevertheless, she conveyed the message clearly: open communication is the only appropriate way to interact with severely ill and dying children. That she wrote more about the children's problems than about how she cared for the children is somewhat unfortunate. Raimbault showed none of the ambiguity that was clearly evident in the other authors and in the work of Anna Freud and her collaborator T. Bergmann (1972). It would have been desirable at the time and also helpful for the sick children if she had formulated her call to talk openly with severely ill and dying children more clearly in her book.

The children's hospital in Paris was the source of another psychotherapy-based article that appeared in the early 1970s (Alby and Alby 1971). I noted earlier how this group distinguished itself by describing carefully how children arrive at their perceptions. They concluded that everything possible should be done in the future to prevent sick children from getting information. The study is characterized by the authors' ambivalence, although, as we will see, they had obviously also studied the literature from the United States and had made substantial progress. They devoted an entire chapter of their extensive study to the development of sick children. They wrote about how impressed they were by the children's ability to observe carefully, and how accurately the children registered the anxieties of those around them. In a section on "Secrets and Communication," they described how the increasing sensitization of the staff made it necessary to change the practice of keeping silent. This was contrary to the French tradition in which the child was to be protected by being excluded, in other words by not receiving information.

They cited the work of Vernick and Karon (1965) and asked whether the insistence on openness therein might not express a different attitude in American medicine. They had two reservations about the attitude of "rejecting the lie." First, the doctors didn't have an exact idea of how long the course of the disease would be, so when they imparted the diagnosis, they were forced to be vague about the future. But it is not clear to me why the authors believed that children couldn't understand this fact. The other point is somewhat more complex; it relates to what Alby and Alby perceived as the American authors' failure to analyze the doctors' real motives. The Americans would simply claim that the children "know" more about their diagnosis than we think and that they are also aware to some extent of their high-risk status. But this doesn't mean that any action is necessary. And so Alby and Alby supported the position Solnit and Green had taken in 1963 that the age of the child, his physical condition, and his family environment must be considered. This is fine in principle, but I mentioned earlier in this chapter that Green (1967) spoke out for honesty several years later, although even then a certain ambivalence could still be perceived. These sorts of reservations lead us to suspect that the French authors wanted to keep an escape hatch open—a phenomenon we can still observe in many doctors to this day when they claim to support openness and honesty but add that there are exceptions in individual cases. Too often, the exceptional cases become the majority!

And so Alby and Alby explained, "Everyone who has tried to discover what children need has agreed that we must avoid two behaviors: we must not keep silent at any price, and we must not maintain a conspiratorial atmosphere in which we avoid all the questions children might ask about their illness."

They concluded that it is necessary to connect the rule of silence about the illness and the way the child lives with the ban on knowledge. This could be accounted for quite naturally by conflicts in emotional development, in particular by the repression of sexual curiosity. To know or not to know is frightening not only because of the significance of the diagnosis or prognosis; it also means a transgression of the permissible: the child does what he has been forbidden to do and thus becomes culpable. Here the two authors' psychoanalytic way of thinking, firmly anchored in the system developed by Sigmund Freud, becomes evident. It isn't surprising that many pediatricians at the time stayed out of this kind of discussion.

In 1974 American child psychoanalyst Shirley B. Lansky described the role she played as part of a pediatric oncology team. In the article, she explained in detail how parents were informed of their children's diagnosis and how she accompanied the parents during therapy. Amazingly, she wrote almost nothing about the children except that many of them developed a phobia of schools. A child psychiatrist's primary concern should actually be the children and not the parents. Another study from the same time dealt only with the parents of sick children (Kirkpatrick et al. 1974). The subject was the phobia of schools, which was a serious problem at that time, in cases where children were not able to find out what was the matter with them. The children were kept in the dark and so were their schoolmates, who usually did have some suspicions. Often they avoided the sick child because they didn't know how to handle this "secret." This problem was of such concern to Lansky (1975) that she published an article on the topic. This is not the place to show how this phobia can be eliminated; suffice to say that it is an important problem we need to keep in mind when caring for sick children and adolescents.

John Spinetta, a psychologist, carried out in-depth studies of the fears of children with leukemia during the second half of the 1970s (Spinetta et al. 1973; Spinetta 1974; Spinetta and Maloney 1975). He found that children with leukemia do not necessarily express their worries and fears openly. But they definitely do have fears that arise from the seriousness of their illness.

Whether these fears can be labeled "fear of death" he considered a question of semantics. He did not mention the possibility of informing the children in these articles. It is apparent that he was not yet sure of the correct course of action. But in his article in *The Child and Death* (1978), edited by Olle J. Sahler, he concluded that openness is the right approach (Spinetta and Maloney 1978). Three years later, his position was unambiguous (Spinetta and Deasy-Spineta 1981a), and he endorsed Vernick and Karon's (1965) view of openness in interactions with children.

Spinetta's name appears often in the literature, especially as the coauthor of publications of the Working Committee on Psychosocial Issues of the International Society of Paediatric Oncology (SIOP, Société Internationale d'Oncologie Pédiatrique). In 1981 he edited, with Patricia Deasy-Spinetta, the important book *Living with Childhood Cancer*; in one chapter, he summarized the development to date of the discussion around informing children and his own research on children with cancer. The final chapter of the book, in which the authors compiled their research results, is about talking with children. All of these results provide evidence that we should be open with children.

The book also includes a valuable article by psychologist R. S. Lazarus about the costs and benefits of denial. He wanted to show that denial is one possible way for a sick person to live with his or her illness. Denial is a human strategy often used to "banish" unpleasant things. Not informing children naturally promotes this strategy. Lazarus clearly stated that denial at the beginning of a serious illness can be a useful strategy while the patient's resources are still insufficient to dealing with the illness adequately. After some time has passed, the patient may be able to confront his problems actively. Lazarus did say that when the patient is confronted with the problem over and over again, denial gets in the way of finally mastering it.

In her wonderful book *The Private Worlds of Dying Children*, Myra Bluebond-Langner (1978) went into all of the essential points of how to interact with severely ill and dying children; the book was discussed earlier, in chapter 9. She began the chapter on interacting with dying children by asserting that the most important question is what we say to children. It is fundamentally similar to dealing with sex: tell them what they want to know, and do it in words they can understand. We can already see that she still felt a certain ambivalence. Bluebond-Langner consistently evaded giving a definitive statement, but at the same time she considered openness to be important. She thought it was not so important *whether* we say something, but *what* we say.

Unfortunately she did not have an unambiguous answer ready, so she was stuck with the approach that was common practice at the time. That does not detract from the value of the book when we consider that it was published in 1978, at a time when many authors were still struggling with the concept of openness.

In her book *In the Shadow of Illness* (Bluebond-Langner 1996), which was published twenty years later, she finally took a clear position. She wrote that parents can manage to hide the truth from their children only for a short time. They will learn over time that this approach has no advantages. She also believed that openness within the family increases as death comes closer. I have already mentioned her excellent publications (2003, 2006) in which she left absolutely no doubt that open communication with sick children is the right way.

In 1982 the publication of Ruprecht Nitschke's working group in Oklahoma City appeared. For the first time, they reported that terminally ill six- to twenty-year-old patients were involved in the decision of whether another treatment using an experimental therapy should be attempted. The prerequisite for this "final-stage conference," as they called it, is of course that those affected know exactly what the issue is. In this context, they cited the work of Vernick and Karon (1965) and Spinetta (1981). They were convinced that the approach suggested by these authors was the right one. They reported on more than forty-three patients and confirmed that no serious problems arose. Children over five had understood the finality of their own death and were able to make rational decisions about how to proceed. It is interesting that all of the parents agreed to this approach, which was disturbing—especially for that time. This is evidence that the working group involved them closely in the children's care from the beginning.

Loretta Kopelman had already concluded by 1978, based on philosophical and ethical considerations, that dying people, both children and adults, should be informed of their clinical situation and should be involved in decisions about treatment. I return to this in the next chapter when I discuss the question of the extent to which children should be involved in such decisions. When Nitschke presented his group's approach to the German Pediatrician's Conference in Tübingen in 1984, he elicited a lot of unease and incredulity. A year later, Nitschke and his collaborators (1985) described the problem of providing psychological care to chronically ill children in the *Monatsschrift Kinderheilkunde*; this article was discussed in detail in chapter 9.

Further support for the concept of open communication appeared the same year as the article from Oklahoma City. L. Slavin and collaborators (1982) showed that children who learn their diagnosis at an early stage of their illness cope with the illness much better than children who find out late and indirectly. They interviewed surviving cancer patients as well as their parents and siblings; most of them advised communicating the diagnosis as early as possible. Many parents who hadn't done so indicated that their lack of courage to communicate openly was a source of many difficulties and burdens during and after treatment. The authors thought that early communication of the diagnosis was also evidence of the frank atmosphere in which the sick child had grown up. Parents who had informed their child against the doctors' advice did not want to give up the approach characterized by openness and honesty that the family had taken up to that point. In his book *Childhood and Death* (1984) published a few years later, E. H. Waechter expressed the opinion that children always find out what is causing their illness, even if a major effort is made to prevent it. In a book edited by Hannelore Wass and Charles A. Corr, various authors expressed the same point of view.

Another book was published in the United States with the title *The Child and Death* (Schowalter et al. 1983). It included a chapter by Melvin Lewis and Dorothy Otnow Lewis about dying children and their families. It is worth quoting them here because they described in a nutshell the doctors' problem, on the one hand, and the children's problem, on the other. They made it clear that there are at least three reasons that a dying child is frightening to a doctor: feelings of incompetence, feelings of failure, and the fear of being confronted with his or her own limitations and mortality. The doctor also has difficulties dealing with the parents' fear, their fury and depression, their displeasure and denial. The situation is complex because dying is a transitional stage and each case seems to be different. At first glance, there does not seem to be any obviously correct way to deal with the child, with his or her family, and with oneself and one's colleagues. A doctor may at first try to protect him- or herself by avoiding the dying child, hiding his or her evasion with various attempts at rationalization. Like the child, the doctor doesn't want to talk about his or her situation or becomes flustered if anyone tries to talk to him or her about it. But the family and the child look to the doctor for understanding, support, and guidance.

There is almost nothing the child or his parents may fear, imagine, feel, or experience that cannot be discussed honestly with them. The basis for such a discussion is a relationship of mutual trust. Children learn especially quickly whom they can trust, and that is the person to whom they will open up. In fact, children sense more clearly what adults can endure than adults sense how well children can adapt. And children behave accordingly. The authors asked how doctors should behave, and they concluded that knowing how children and parents react to death and dying under various circumstances and what they understand provides us with a foundation for a solid clinical procedure.

The necessity of being open and honest with sick children could hardly be expressed more clearly. The authors emphasized that parents must always be involved and that the contact person for the child must be clearly designated. In addition, all members of the team must be kept adequately informed in the same way. But just for the record—the discussion continued even after the publication of this book.

There are few studies that ask to what extent children understand a severe illness and its treatment. A British working group did pose this question, keeping in mind that, in contrast to before, children with cancer had to adapt to living with a severe illness (Kendrick et al. 1987). They studied twenty-five children between the ages of two and eleven in connection with three inter-related questions:

- How do children with cancer understand their illness and its treatment?
- How does this understanding (or misunderstanding) develop?
- What significance does the correct understanding have for the sick child?

In summary, the findings were that children with cancer learned about their illness in a variety of ways, through both verbal and nonverbal information. Particularly in the beginning, they are in an alert phase during which they absorb a lot of information. Later, some children may exclude the absorption of further information through repression or denial. Much more often, however, children collect information continually. Since they get information from a variety of sources, it is particularly important that these sources be unambiguous and honest, not contradictory.

Many children make impressive advances in development, as other authors have already described (Waechter 1971; Spinetta 1974; Bluebond-Langner 1978). It is interesting to observe that they often display a certain regression in their behavior at the same time. Children of very different ages are able to understand different stages of their illness and its treatment. Even the young children in the study could understand the significance for them of concrete aspects of life in the hospital as well as the dichotomy of good and bad indications in the course of their illness. The children learn a lot through practical experience, so the first time a certain procedure is carried out constitutes basic information. Play is also important for dealing with the illness. The authors conclude that how well the child understands or perhaps misunderstands his or her illness plays a major role. Especially in the latter case, children may experience a great deal of fear, especially if they are quieter, more withdrawn, or younger and therefore not able to clarify the situation using targeted questioning. So the outcome of this study is a further plea for exchanging information openly with sick children.

In 1987 Mark A. Chesler and Oscar A. Barbarin published the monograph *Childhood Cancer and the Family: Meeting the Challenge of Stress and Support*, about interacting with children and adolescents with cancer; the year before, they had written about parents' approach to dealing with their child (Chesler et al. 1986). They too supported openness; they paid particular attention to the problems of adolescents. They pointed to an article by P. Lang and C. Mitrowski that had appeared in 1981, in which the authors noted that it can be beneficial for older children and adolescents if they are treated and cared for in an institution specifically designed for children with cancer. There patients are able to make friends with similarly affected children of the same age, which is extremely helpful in coping with their situation. These statements contrast markedly with the ideas of the early 1970s, when an institution of that kind was rejected as being problematic at best. With regard to the question of how open we should be with children, they referred to the work of Vernick and Karon (1965), whose conclusions they wholeheartedly supported.

American pediatric oncologist Edwin Forman and philosopher Rosalin Ekman Ladd published a study in 1989 about how far we should go in telling children the truth in the face of medical uncertainty and disagreement about how to proceed in individual cases. In this outstanding study, the authors investigated in great detail how disagreements arise among doctors and what we should conclude from this. Uncertainty about the right way to proceed is not unusual in medicine, and all prospective doctors must learn to cope with it. There are two sources of disagreement. On the one hand, there can be different opinions about certain facts; that is, doctors are often in disagreement about the correct interpretation of existing data. On the other hand, there are differing approaches and moral concepts among doctors.

Knowing this, doctors have to make up their minds about how they will arrive at their own ideas and the recommendations for their patients that will be based on them. They must then share this knowledge with their patients so that they too can reflect on their own approach and moral concepts in order to reach the right decision. The authors' main concern here was informing the parents of severely ill children. I mention it because I believe the process described is also valid for dealing with the children themselves, and I know from many personal conversations with Forman that he is of the same opinion.

At the same time, the American philosopher D. Brock (1989) was looking critically at children's competence in making decisions. After ample consideration, he concluded that there may be a lot of variability among children but that it is safe to assume that children under the age of nine are not competent to understand the consequences of their illness and therefore there is no need to tell them the truth. I discuss this and other studies in more detail when I address the subject of children's decisionmaking abilities. My goal here is to make clear that toward the end of the 1980s, the discussion slowly closed in on the fundamental problem of whether and to what extent we should give information to children.

This is demonstrated in another study from the same year, in which John Graham-Pole and his collaborators (1989) performed a retrospective analysis of the communication between dying children and their siblings. Seventy-seven mothers filled out questionnaires with forty-nine items. The authors studied the factors that influenced the extent and success of open communication among the parents, the dying child, and the child's siblings. They had acted on the assumption that children over four with a life-threatening illness have a premonition of their death. Age at the time of death was 12.4±4.9 years on average, and the length of illness was 4.1±5.1 years on average. Children over twelve spoke more often about their deaths than younger children, and siblings of children who suspected they would soon die also knew about the situation early on.

Through their responses, forty-one of the seventy-seven mothers enabled the authors to find out to what extent talking about their own death was helpful to the children. Twenty-four mothers (58.5%) indicated that such conversations were helpful, while the remaining mothers were less positive or even negative. The two most important factors that were assessed positively were, first, that the child was at home during the terminal stage and, second, that the child had a primary contact person. Other positive factors were the extent of communication, the individual points discussed, and whether the actual process of death was discussed. Religious belief too had a positive influence, and it was especially helpful for the child when it included extensive and detailed information about death and dying. It is interesting to note that according to the mothers' responses, the two factors found to be positive for the sick children had an equally positive influence on siblings, although they were not helpful in exactly the same way. It was obviously not easy for the mothers to evaluate the situation of the healthy siblings.

Pediatric oncologists are familiar with the fact that parents concentrate much more on the sick children and don't pay as much attention to healthy siblings. The dialogues with the sick children may also have been more intense, and this may have led the mothers retrospectively to assume that the conversations were not so important for the healthy siblings. The results discussed in detail in the article are worthwhile. It is clear that the authors valued open communication a great deal. They determined that appropriate communication is at least as important for the survivors as it is for the dying children. Siblings should be encouraged to play an important role in preparing the sick child for death (Chesler and Barbarin 1987). Active listening and support require courage, experience, time, and patience as well as trial and error. The family dialogue should begin as early as possible; fortunately, the siblings and parents can continue it beyond the child's death. This study is certainly worth reading. With the phrase "trial and error," the authors advocated engaging in dialogue over and over again; this includes being willing to make mistakes.

An article by psychologists Carol J. Claflin and Oscar A. Barbarin was published in 1991. Using an earlier study as a starting point (Chesler and Barbarin 1986), they wanted to investigate whether sick children were better protected if they were told less. The earlier study had determined that many parents of children with cancer believed that young children don't understand the diagnosis and prognosis of their illness, with the result that the young children received much less information from their parents than the older children. Many parents also believe the proverb "What I don't know won't hurt me" applies to their children. The theory is that children who know nothing or almost nothing will have many fewer worries and fears if they are spared negative information. Logically, the young children should worry much less than the older children, who found out more from their parents. Claflin and Barbarin came to the conclusion that this assumption is wrong and that the level of anxiety is just as high for the uninformed children as it is for the others. They also assumed that children know more than adults think. It would be much better to inform the children in order to make coping with the situation easier. In addition, Claflin and Barbarin concluded that the methods employed by psychology are insufficient for analyzing children's level of understanding and how they manage it.

In 1991 the psychologist D. Bearson published a book with the title *They Never Want to Tell You—Children Talk about Cancer,* in which he wrote plainly that we should explain everything to children as early as possible in the course of their illness. He cited L. Slavin and his collaborators (1982), who had shown years earlier that early and open communication helps children deal with their illness. Bearson pointed out how important it is for children to talk about their illness and to give them an opportunity to tell stories and to confront their illness in a dialogue with their caregivers. The book includes eight stories told to him by sick children and an extensive chapter on themes that children like to tell stories about. I recommend the book above all to those who refuse to believe that we need to open a dialogue with children and continue it until their death.

Other authors at the time came to similar conclusions; they determined that children should be thoroughly informed about their illness and its treatment. Only the terminally ill, however, want to be involved in deciding how to proceed, while children in the early stages of cancer are satisfied with what the adults decide for them (Ellis and Leventhal 1993). This is easy to explain, since early in the illness children usually do not have the experience needed to make decisions. They are still overwhelmed by the negative diagnosis. Closer to the end of life, things look very different.

In London in 1993 Ann Goldmann and Deborah Christie published a remarkable study in which they investigated whether and how children with cancer talk with their families about their own deaths. The two authors assumed that a consensus had developed in the meantime in the literature—in support of open dialogue with children. In 1989 they administered a questionnaire to members of a team in pediatric hematology and oncology at the Hospital for Sick Children. The authors administered the questionnaire to team members who had cared for a dying child one week after the child's death. They learned that when it became clear that death was approaching,

the situation was discussed openly with the parents. All team members encouraged the parents to be open and honest. During that year, thirty-nine
children between the ages of ten weeks and sixteen years old died; most of
the children died at home. Since the literature at the time reported that only
children older than three had any understanding of death, the younger children were excluded from the analysis. Twenty-six of the thirty-one children
were told that they had experienced a relapse. An analysis of statements by
the team members who knew the family and the child best resulted in four
groups with regard to the "level of knowledge":

- The child and his family knew death would occur soon. Both sides
  were aware of the other's knowledge. Only in one case, however, was
  there an open discussion (n=6 of 31).
- The child never articulated the concept of death. The nurses, however, had the feeling that the child knew about it but didn't want to
  talk about it (n=9 of 31).
- The child never articulated the concept of death, and the nurses had
  the feeling that the child also didn't know about it (n=9 of 31).
- Unknown (n=7 of 31).

The study also shows that the length of illness is positively correlated with
open communication.

Next, twenty-two experienced team members (doctors, nurses, and social
workers) who had spoken in support of open communication were questioned.
The team members assumed that a certain percentage of the children had
spoken openly about their death; this percentage varied between 10 percent
and 80 percent (median: 45%). This result is astounding, but on second
thought, perhaps not so surprising. The parents had truly spoken openly
with their child in only a single case. In contrast to this, the team members
assumed they had done so in an average of 50 percent of the cases. It is interesting to note that one doctor cited 80 percent, while two of the three social
workers assessed the situation much more realistically (10 and 15 percent).

Goldmann and Christie believed that the study confirmed their impression that doctors are convinced that openness is the right approach in providing care but that in fact few parents act accordingly. This study demonstrates strikingly how team members' assessments of the situation were in
general completely incorrect. In the authors' opinion, they had not recognized
how much more difficult it is in practice to talk with a child about his or her

impending death. Pediatricians talk much more with parents than with the children and like to leave the task of talking with the children to the parents. The authors appealed to professional staff (in particular doctors and other caregivers) to pursue the matter more energetically and to realize how difficult open communication is for parents. For this reason, it is their responsibility to improve their own competencies in this area and to help the parents. Although the number of children studied was small, the results throw an interesting light on the situation in 1993. We must ask ourselves whether the situation is so different today.

In 1994 the English nurse Edward Purssell added his voice to the discussion (Purssell 1994). He referred primarily to the publication by Nitschke and collaborators (1982) and found that children always know what the issue is but that parents often hesitate to talk with their children. Nurses and other caregivers should not allow this fact to keep children from getting the treatment they deserve. They should make it clear to parents that their children know most of what there is to know and that doctors and nurses are not prepared to lie to the children. He too believed that children can and should make decisions themselves. Purssell's work clarifies a fact that doctors like to forget: it is the nurses and other care providers who care for the children all day long and who perceive their needs much better, since they talk with the children and their parents often. They are probably the ones who have the biggest problem with keeping silent and the resulting charade because they have to do it all day long. Until the 1990s, the nursing staff and other caregivers seldom spoke up.

In 1996 American pediatrician John D. Lantos posed the question directly in the title of his article "Should We Always Tell Children the Truth?" He begins by noting that "truth-telling" is a curious cultural artifact. America is especially preoccupied with it, and it plays a central role in the consideration of how a reasonable relationship between patient and doctor looks. Every deviation from "truth telling" is viewed as a relapse into paternalism. Lantos thinks that this should demystify illness and that truth is the first step toward clarity.

Later in the article, Lantos observes that even the strongest supporters of providing full information realize that they have to fall back on parents in the case of very young children. And since very young children cannot decide for themselves, the arguments in support of providing information must be based to a large extent on morality. He writes, "We tell the truth to children, it seems, not to empower them, or gain their cooperation and achieve good outcomes, or to make them aware of our conflicts of interest, but simply because the truth is good." And: "The doctors might gain a sort of moral self-aggrandizement by telling the truth. This would be partly selfish. Their consciences would be eased. They would not have to suffer from participating in a deception, or question whether the conventional moral wisdom was always correct. The hospital lawyers would be happy. Telling the truth is always good for risk-management, although it is a fact that we have to question how much it really empowers patients."

It could be, Lantos continues, that truth provides some kind of advantage for the child. In his opinion, however, this assumption rests only on the doctors' rather utilitarian hope that patients feel better when they know the truth. Doctors don't consider whether patients are able to cope with so much truth. Lantos believes that truth can also be devastating, as he writes: "One problem with doctors and truth-telling is that we're not very good story tellers. We cannot imagine medical scenarios as real tragedies. We cannot imagine ourselves as shamans, or healers. We seem to be having trouble remembering what it means to be a doctor, or seeing the connections between what we call morality and risk-management, between the narrow view of the truth-telling which turns doctors into providers and patients into clients and the larger problems in medicine today."

Lantos writes that sick people need affection, concern, and comfort rather than facts. He asks whether our truth shouldn't be some form of religious, spiritual, or artistic interaction with the patient that is different from what we understand in our society as truth. Lantos closes, "I can't imagine how I would behave if my daughter and granddaughter were dying of AIDS, whether I would choose the brutal truth or a comforting lie. But I do know that, whatever I chose, I would not want a doctor judging the morality of my decision. I would want a doctor who could listen to me, comfort me, hug me, cry with me, or just be with me, but not one who would judge me. Sometimes, perhaps, even in America, the best medicine might still be a comforting lie."

After the 1970s and especially the 1980s, when we can observe a clear trend in support of honesty, this article seems almost like a throwback. I have quoted Lantos so extensively here because he expresses the position opposed to truthfulness so clearly, a position that still receives support today. The most important part of the article is the conclusion, in which the author describes the two alternatives he sees: the doctor with the brutal truth or the doctor who does everything we (including myself) should expect a good and helpful doctor to do and also utilizes the comforting lie.

I will say more about this later, but I emphasize at this point that these are not the only two alternatives. The first doctor, the one who in the author's eyes employs only brutal truth and otherwise has nothing to offer, is not a good doctor and thus not an alternative. But we are not talking about revealing a brutal truth, we are talking about a doctor's professional conduct that includes everything Lantos expects from a good doctor. We are talking about a relationship of mutual trust that people who are dying need. And part of that relationship is honesty and confidence that no one is lying. This is the only way to avoid leaving the dying person alone in his desperate situation. It is amazing that this does not seem to be an issue for Lantos. And he also does not see it as relevant that children can cope better with their illnesses if they are well informed, although this was demonstrated by Slavin and his collaborators in 1982. I am certain that the author himself does possess all the qualities that he expects a good doctor to have. It seems to me that his arguments, which have the ring of empathy, are there to cloak his fears of the open approach.

The second book by Myra Bluebond-Langner was published the same year as Lantos's article (1996). She writes that it makes no sense to withhold the truth from children because it can only be successful for a short time; parents would soon learn that it isn't worth it to take that approach. If we compare the explanations of Lantos and Bluebond-Langner, we get the impression that they come from two different worlds; their views could not be more antithetical.

One year later, the SIOP Working Committee on Psychosocial Issues in Pediatric Oncology published a guideline on how to communicate a diagnosis in the right way (Masera et al. 1997). The question of *whether* the diagnosis should be communicated to the sick child is not even asked; it is taken as self-evident that it should be communicated. Instead, sensitive recommendations for doctors are formulated that are certainly helpful, if they are read. The most important statement is made at the beginning:

> Providing information is not a one-time occurrence; it is a process that offers the possibility again and again to respond to the needs of the children and their parents.

All oncologists, whether they treat adults or children, should frame this sentence and hang it above their desks, because it is true that this process begins with the first meeting with the patient and ends with his or her death (or today, fortunately, often with their final cure).

In 1998 a Japanese group published similar guidelines, although they were intended for cancer patients in general, not just for children (Okamura et al. 1998). They leave no doubt that medical staff should be open with the patients and that the goal is to improve communication. The authors report that open interactions with patients are still fundamentally difficult for Japanese doctors. Since there were still no guidelines for "informed consent" in any of the hospitals or universities in Japan in 1996, they applied themselves to developing some. The published version in English is a revised version of the original resolution. The paper contains many good suggestions for doctors who want to interact in a satisfactory way with cancer patients. I mention one section here because it illustrates clearly what Lantos may have meant by "brutal truth." They write, "Patients are sometimes told, 'You have advanced cancer and there is nothing I can do. There is no effective treatment in your case.' Such a cruel attitude presented by the physician causes loss of hope, anger, resignation and a sense of alienation in patients. Physicians should recognize that they can generate both hope and despair in patients by their verbal expression or attitude. Physicians should present other positive features, including supportive care, instead of abandoning a patient with such a statement."

I think that we can without hesitation characterize this kind of behavior on the part of physicians as harsh, and the Japanese authors rejected it unambiguously. Saying *"I can't do anything more for you"* means that you intend to abandon the patient to his fate.

This is apparent in the book by Christoph Schmeling-Kludas that was published in 1988. In Germany, rejecting this kind of approach had already gained acceptance in the medical treatment of adults by this time; his excellent description of this issue and his summary of the literature are intended to adapt the doctor-patient relationship to modern ideas within the framework of hospital routine.

In 1999 in the journal *Pediatrics,* the American Academy of Pediatrics took a position on the question of whether we should tell children with AIDS the truth about their illness. It too advocates telling children with chronic illnesses the truth. This is true for children with HIV infections as well, at least for schoolchildren over the age of five or six, even though their prognosis is particularly uncertain.

In the same year, further guidelines from the SIOP Working Committee on Psychosocial Issues in Pediatric Oncology were published (Masera et al. 1999) on assistance to terminally ill children. Here too, open communication is taken as a given without going into details. In a long letter to the editor, Nitschke (2000) comments on the guidelines. He welcomes them in principle but sees some flaws. In his view, the link between age and providing information remains too vague, and the insistence that hope always be maintained is too general. He also thinks some other concepts are not defined clearly enough. In a brief response, the authors of the guidelines basically accept the critique. They point out that Nitschke's comments do not contradict the guidelines, which had to merge various realities since the authors came from various countries with ethnic, cultural, and linguistic differences. It is readily understandable that it is not easy to find an international consensus on this complex topic (Masera and Jancovic 2000).

In 2000, an issue of the highly respected *Journal of Clinical Oncology* appeared on the subject "The Art of Oncology: When the Tumor Is Not the Target." One short article in this issue was entitled "Tell the Children" (Hilden et al. 2000). The authors describe two scenarios for a dying child that differ considerably. The parents of a six-year-old girl insisted on the strategy of denial. Members of the treatment team disagreed, since they recognized that the child was afraid, but they accepted the parents' decision. No one talked openly with her about her death. Well before the child's death, it became clear that, despite the parents' strategy, her eight-year-old sister realized her sister would die. In the second case, the parents of an eight-year-old boy behaved completely differently. From the very beginning, everything was discussed openly with the boy, including the fact that there were no further therapeutic options after the third recurrence of his leukemia and that he would die. His sister was informed too, and in contrast to the first family, she was included in plans for the funeral.

The authors argue that the parents' course of action in the first case was bad for both children, the sick child and her healthy sister. They were unable to convince the parents to change their approach, although some team members thought that with more time and information, they might have succeeded. The authors compare the two cases as an argument in favor of honesty. In an editorial, P. M. Anderson (2000) confirms that honesty is the best policy toward children of all ages. He also points out how important it is for the caregivers to share the burden, something that is apparent in the case histories. Ruprecht Nitschke and his collaborators (2001) also comment on this article in a letter. Here too they criticize missing and vague statements, but their criticism is not a fundamental one. Nitschke and his collaborators also summarize the basic principles of their approach (2000). They renewed the plea for honesty that was expressed clearly in their earlier publications.

That same year, Phyllis R. Silvermann's notable book *Never Too Young to Know: Death in Children's Lives* was published in the United States. In this book, Silvermann considers all the aspects of death with which children can be confronted. Therefore only one chapter—a very worthwhile one—is devoted to the child's own death. Using many examples, she clarifies for the reader how communication with dying children can vary, how helpful a religious affiliation can be for the parents, and what may confront parents in this situation. This chapter is also a plea for honesty.

In 2004, A. G. Tuckett, an Australian nurse, published a survey article in which she listed the arguments in favor of honesty as well as the corresponding counterarguments. This article does not refer specifically to children but instead deals with the general issue of truth. According to the author, doing anything other than telling the truth contradicts the principle of patient autonomy. At the same time, the truth enables the patient to cope with his or her situation. She cites articles from the literature that express the chief counterargument—that it is necessary to tell the truth within the current commercialized doctor-patient relationship, but that there is also an adequate argument for paternalistic lying in order to protect the patient. She concludes that in each case the doctor must find out what the patient and his family want. This article is more or less a step backward, but Tuckett is attempting to summarize and comment on the arguments for and against openness that had been employed in the literature, and she does not take a clear position herself.

In the same year, an article by a Swedish working group with the title "Talking about Death with Children Who Have Severe Malignant Disease" appeared in the *New England Journal of Medicine* (Kreicbergs et al. 2004). The authors contacted 561 parents of 368 children who had become ill with cancer under the age of seventeen and had died between 1992 and 1997. Of the group, 449 parents responded and filled out a questionnaire. The main questions were:

- Did you talk about death with your child at any time?
    a. If the answer was no: Do you wish that you had?
    b. If the answer was yes: Do you wish that you had not?
- When do you think your child realized that he or she was going to die?

The authors tried to measure the extent of parents' anxiety and depression with additional questions. The results were as follows:

- 147 parents (34%) talked with their child about death; in other words, two-thirds of the responding parents had not done so.
- None of the 147 parents who had talked with their child regretted doing so.
- 69 of the 258 parents (27%) who did not talk to their child regretted this later, while the other 189 (73%) did not.
- 191 parents (46%) never had the feeling that their child suspected they were going to die.
- 91 parents (22%) reported that it was not until the last week before death occurred that they had the feeling their child suspected something. 48 parents (11%) reported that the child had no suspicions until about two to four weeks before his or her death. Only 39 parents (9%) already noticed more than three months before their child's death that he or she suspected something.

The authors then carried out extensive statistical analyses of the characteristics of the parent groups that had behaved in different ways; the results do not play a role here because they don't contribute to solving the real problem. If we consider everything that has been reported up to now in the existing literature about dealing with truth and if we consider the conclusions most authors of research studies reached during the 1990s, then the results of this study are alarming. Even in a modern Western country, only a third of parents talked with their severely ill children about their death, and half of the parents were sure that their children suspected nothing. It is not surprising that that the percentage of parents who communicated was greater in the group where the children suspected something.

It amazed me that Kreicbergs and her colleagues don't really express the conclusions that the results of their study seem to demand. The only comment they make is in the article's final paragraph: "Parents who seek advice—'Should I, or should I not, talk with my child about death?'—might benefit from knowing that no parent in this study regretted having talked about it. In addition, the fact that many parents who had sensed that their child was aware of his or her imminent death later regretted not having talked about death emphasizes the clear responsibility of health care workers to help parents respond to the wants and needs of a terminally ill child."

It is astonishing that this statement is so weak, since by this time the need for openness was widely acknowledged. This tentative quality of the article can possibly be ascribed to the fact that its source is an institute for cancer epidemiology and not a hospital. It is clear from reading the article that there was too little communication with the dying children; this is probably not their fault, since they are all theoreticians and obviously not involved in patient care. I am also not sure whether the authors include doctors and nurses under the label "health care worker"—which would be correct—or whether they include only other professional groups such as social workers, psychologists, and social pedagogues. It is surprising that the authors don't cite the article by Graham-Pole and collaborators, since they had also interviewed mothers in 1989 and had taken a clear position on the importance and necessity of open communication.

Shortly thereafter, a commentary by the American pediatric oncologist Lawrence Wolfe appeared in the same volume of the journal (2004). He first recognizes that in many cases a point is reached when we have to be honest ("when everyone sees the elephant in the room"). But he then declares that there is plenty of evidence that even young children understand the existence of death and that attitudes toward death and its meaning follow a powerful series of developmental steps. And there is also evidence, he continues, that it is beneficial for families if they can speak with their children about their approaching death. His conclusion—in 2004!—is formulated in such a weak way that it leaves much to be desired: "The study by Kreicbergs et al. uses new statistical models and a large population to give a clear message about the intimate emotional experience of parents with a dying child. Pediatric oncologists can now say, not only from their own experience but also from the experience of the hundreds of parents in this study, that no parent regretted talking to his or her child about death. If the child appeared to be aware of impending death (and I believe most such children are), this investigation may help those of us who care for the breaking heart as well."

Wolf is really just repeating the wording of Kreicbergs and her colleagues in their conclusions, and there is not a word in his commentary about the fact that only a third of the parents talked with their children. Wolf also does not offer any clear recommendations for the right course of action. Are we still seeing the same ambivalence we have seen so often before? The statistics offer some information about the parents who did talk with their children. I agree that the article provides evidence that parents don't have to be afraid they will come to regret having spoken with their children. Still, in the year 2004, this is paltry stuff. Any pediatric oncologist who has had experience with parents who spoke openly with their children could have come to this conclusion; we didn't really need these statistics. However, I concede that in the field of medicine today, we usually only believe something if it is supported by statistics. This is a message that might have been new twenty or thirty years ago, but not today.

What both the article and the commentary show clearly in the end is that many pediatricians in 2004 are still not prepared to take a firm position and help children receive fair treatment. It is interesting to note that neither the authors nor the commentator mention the article by a British team that had appeared in 1993 (Goldman and Christie 1993); it portrayed the problems clearly, and their conclusions were much clearer, to the point of being unambiguous. The result of all this is that many children still die in isolation. They have to cope with dying alone because pediatricians do not give parents the support that Goldman and Christie (1993) insisted on, simply because they still find it difficult.

It isn't surprising, then, that two letters to the editor about the article by the Swedish working group clearly take a more or less negative position (Davies 2005; Tanvetyanon 2005). Two-thirds of the parents had not talked with their child, clearly the majority. Open information is pointless for children, as opposed to adults, because children don't need it in order to finish something that is unfinished. In their answer to the two letters, the Swedish team confirms that their article says little about the consequences of their findings (Kreicbergs et al. 2005). They emphasize that deciding whether we should speak openly with a particular child must ultimately depend on personal sensitivity, communicative abilities, and clinical experience. I must emphasize again how regrettable I find it that such a feeble discussion of a topic so important for sick children was carried on in the most respected medical journal in the world as late as 2004 and 2005. It certainly cannot help doctors who are insecure in this regard to change their behavior and begin talking with children; severely ill and dying children and adolescents will continue to be abandoned in their distress.

There were others who discussed the Swedish article in the same year (Hurwitz et al. 2004). One important point in their view is that none of the parents who talked about death with their child regretted it. They go one step further by pointing out that a substantial consensus had developed in the meantime that children with a life-threatening illness should be fully informed. They also note that there is still a lot of resistance to this approach, above all from parents. The authors believe that the treatment team should tell parents that they will not tell the child an untruth if he or she asks directly about their prognosis. They give many good suggestions about how to handle a dying child's situation. They believe that information for parents about the possible death of the child should begin early and be continuous, and that this approach will help alleviate suffering at the end of life. I would have preferred that this discussion be part of the Swedish group's article, which would also have given that article more impact.

Another article that was published the same year, "Silence Is Not Golden: Communicating with Children Dying from Cancer" (Beale et al. 2005), had no connection to the article by the Swedish group. Its authors take a clear position and give helpful suggestions on how to handle the difficult but necessary task of talking with a child about death. In conclusion, they write, "Uncertainty is a major psychological burden both for the children and adults with serious illnesses. . . . Thus it is incumbent on those caring for children who are seriously ill to frequently assess their concerns. Caregivers of dying children must often acknowledge their own emotional pain so it does not become an obstacle to open communication. Avoiding discussion of dying for fear of depressing or frightening a child is a counterproductive strategy, which is not borne out by data." It would be difficult to find a better articulation of why open communication is so essential.

An article that appeared in the same year under the direction of Chris Feudtner from Philadelphia, although otherwise impressive, shows that the requirement that children should be openly informed had still not gained general acceptance (Kang et al. 2005). The article, which focuses on chronically ill and dying children, is substantial in both length and content. The authors discuss many aspects of care at the end of life in an informative way. In a short section on "truth telling," they note that most decisions in pediatrics are based on the well-being of children. But they believe that this situation involves a conflict between truth and denial, as another source put it (Tuckett 2004). They believe that there is too little information on the positive impact of open communication with dying children. However, they refer to the statement by the American Academy of Pediatrics (1999), according to which HIV patients cope with their illness better when they know how matters stand. In the end, these authors too support advising parents to inform their children honestly, especially if they ask repeatedly.

Conclusion

In this chapter we retraced the development of communication with severely ill and dying children and adolescents on the basis of the existing literature, a development that apparently is not yet finished. At its beginning was lack of communication; the goal was to protect children from the unpleasant truth. In the 1950s pediatric oncology was the first branch of pediatric and adolescent medicine to begin to face this complex of problems, although many other illnesses could be fatal. It may have been the deadly threat that hovers over every child with cancer that sensitized oncologists. In the 1950s and 1960s, children often died soon after diagnosis, leaving little time for in-depth communication with them. Only as children began to survive longer did doctors and nurses confront the problem of having to converse with them. In the beginning, statements were characterized by great uncertainty. The idea that children didn't want to know anything was rather comforting. But a certain ambivalence began to intrude into this comfortable state of affairs, and we often catch a glimpse of this in the texts.

In 1965, at a time when almost all children with cancer died, the seminal article by Vernick and Karon was published. It depicted the necessary course of action with amazing clarity and provided supporting evidence based on personal experience. The two authors insisted that we must inform children and that we should never lie. This article should have changed everything; it should have banished lying from the hospital. Admittedly, almost nothing changed at first. In the years that followed, the pendulum swung back and forth; even today there is no agreement, although the recommendation that we should be open with children is gaining the upper hand, since other approaches only lead to difficulties.

The article by the Swedish working group that appeared in the respected *New England Journal of Medicine* in 2004, as well as the letters to the editor and the editorial that followed, demonstrate clearly that there is still substantial resistance to practicing openness. Comments are often still ambivalent, and daily interactions with sick children in many places in the world are probably still ambivalent too. I know from personal experience that many a doctor expresses the opinion that informing children is a fundamental responsibility, yet these doctors have many arguments up their sleeves to explain why it shouldn't be done in this or that individual case. And since there is no doubt that it is always difficult—for me as well—to talk with a child about the fact that he or she is dying, it isn't hard to find a pretext for avoiding the conversation. If we are not fundamentally convinced of the soundness of the premise that we must not lie, we will find these pretexts over and over again, to the great disadvantage of the children and their families. We have many instances of this in the meantime, and I have cited them thoroughly enough.

In closing, I would point to a recent article from the United States that uses a different approach to document how important communication with children is. J. W. Mack and her collaborators (2005) interviewed 146 parents of children who died between 1990 and 1999. The goal of the study was to find out how parents evaluated the quality of care in the end-of-life period and what factors were linked to high quality. A bivariate analysis produced the following results. A high quality rating was associated with:

- the parents' perception that the primary oncologist had transmitted bad news in a sensitive and caring way
- clear information about what to expect at the end of life
- a sense of trust in the primary oncologist
- a feeling of preparedness for the circumstances surrounding the child's death
- direct communication between the primary oncologist and the child when the parents felt it was appropriate and agreed

These points were also confirmed in the multivariate analysis.

In the discussion at the end of this article, Mack and her coauthors remark that the type of communication with their child that parents valued most highly is seldom taught at universities and in training programs. But they still make the claim that there are no scientific studies of conversations with children at the end of their lives. I hope the discussion in this chapter has given the reader a different impression. These authors cite only the article by Kreicbergs and collaborators (2004); its deficiencies have been discussed at length in the course of this book. The articles by Vernick and Karon (1965), Nitschke and collaborators (1986, 1985), and Graham-Pole and collaborators (1989), just to name a few examples, are not mentioned at all.

One gets the impression in reading the article that Mack and her coauthors are truly amazed at their findings with regard to communication with children, and they judge them to be valuable. To substantially improve the care of children, they recommend stimulating doctors' understanding for the communication needs of families and children during medical school and improving their training in this area. I should mention that the authors also asked fifty-two doctors which factors they considered most important for provision of care. In contrast to parents, the doctors cited biomedical factors such as pain or the length of the hospital stay at the end of life and not the quality of communication. In the final analysis, this isn't surprising, since quality of communication is usually not taught in medical schools.

CHAPTER ELEVEN

Decisions at the End of Life

Not all cancer treatments for children and adolescents are successful. Even today we see in just under a third of cases that the patient's life cannot be saved with conventional means—in other words, means employed up to now. In this kind of situation completely new questions arise, and both doctor and patient, and in the case of children parents as well, must deal with them. One of these problems is the question of whether a child must agree to an experimental therapy or whether this is solely the responsibility of parents. An entire chapter is devoted to this topic because it is so closely related to the issue of openness and providing information to children and adolescents.

According to German law, parents must always agree to any treatment of patients who are minors. The only exceptions are emergencies when the parents cannot be reached or when they aren't able to agree for other reasons—inability to understand, for example. In such a case the doctor has to decide whether it is an emergency and he or she cannot wait for consent from a parent or guardian. An exception can also be made if parents do not agree to a vital treatment, as has often happened in the past with members of the Jehovah's Witnesses who refuse a blood transfusion for their children. Again, the doctor must decide whether there is an emergency that calls for a lifesaving blood transfusion. If there is, he or she can proceed with the transfusion without the parents' consent. Under certain circumstances, he or she has to involve the courts—when parents refuse chemotherapy for a child with cancer, for example. The situation in pediatrics is different from that in adult medicine, where a patient can always refuse a lifesaving therapy. But children do not belong to their parents, and according to the Basic Law for the Federal Republic of Germany the state must make sure that children are not harmed—even by their own parents.

There are situations, however, in which the agreement of a minor is a prerequisite—in clinical drug trials, for example. In these cases, we use the word *assent* instead of the usual *consent*. There are certain medical specialties too, such as adolescent gynecology, where the law gives minors, people not yet or only to a limited extent contractually competent, a degree of autonomy. The consulting physician is not required to inform parents in every situation. Prevailing opinion tends increasingly to require that children and adolescents receive adequate information about what is happening to them and that they be granted a certain freedom of choice depending on their age.

Whether children and adolescents should be involved in decisions about therapy is the subject of this final chapter. Does there come a time when we should refrain from further attempts at therapy, in other words discontinue therapy once and for all? Should another experimental therapy be attempted? Since the publication of the article by Nitschke and his collaborators in Oklahoma City (1977), we can no longer ignore this problem in pediatric oncology. The authors reported on their experiences with what they refer to as the "final-stage conference." They talked with twenty children and their parents about the fact that their cancers could no longer be cured with conventional methods, so the doctors offered an experimental therapy. Three of the children were six or seven years old. All of the children were able to understand their situation and made a decision.

The authors based their approach on the work of Karon (1973), who insisted that doctors should discuss problems openly with their young cancer patients and their families. This should still be the case when the illness is in an advanced stage and death has become unavoidable. Karon and Vernick had already described this kind of approach in principle in 1965 (Vernick and Karon 1965). The authors retrace in detail the history of nine of the twenty patients who took part in a conference. Sixteen of the children were in agreement with their parents about further treatment, and four made a decision different from the one their parents favored. Eight of the nine children made their decision independently of their parents. In no case did either parents or children regret having been told the truth.

Misgivings about this approach were expressed right away in a letter to the editor (Shumway et al. 1983); supposedly this approach took away the children's hope. Nitschke (2000) commented later in another context, pointing out that the author of the letter had equated "hope" with "hope for survival." This kind of hope is unrealistic in the case of a dying child, and survival must be replaced by another perspective. Nitschke's view is correct. For much too long, medicine argued that we should never take hope away from a dying patient (including the hope of survival) by openly explaining his or her situation to him. Most dying people—children included—realize at some point that this hope has become unrealistic. Of course in this situation we should not take from the patient the hope of experiencing certain things that are important to him or her (confirmation or communion, a visit to an aunt or uncle, or a particular trip).

Unfortunately, the 1977 article by Nitschke and his collaborators appeared in a journal on child psychology and therefore was mostly overlooked by pediatricians. Although the Oklahoma authors later published related articles in pediatric journals in the United States and Germany, skepticism toward this approach has not yet disappeared even today (Nitschke et al. 1985, 1986, 2000). A discussion about this issue didn't really get going until the turn of the twenty-first century. That the authors developed clear ideas about this approach is important, since these ideas can serve as a basis for scientific evaluation. Together with my collaborators, I developed and published what was in principle a comparable approach based on never lying (Niethammer and Hoffmeister 1983; Niethammer 1992, 1995a, 1995b, 1998, 2008; Schreiber-Gollwitzer 2002). Since our approach follows fewer specific rules, it may be harder to evaluate scientifically. In the final analysis, though, both working groups agree that children should always be involved, even in the most difficult decisions.

A working group of pediatricians and representatives of other professional bodies involved in the care of seriously ill children met in the United States in 1994. For three days, they developed fundamental ideas about how to care for seriously ill children and involve them in decisionmaking. A summary of the results was published in *Pediatrics*, the preeminent American journal in the field (Fleischman et al. 1994). The participants in the conference agreed that up to that point there were no clear ideas on this issue. The article deals with almost all aspects of this complex of problems in exemplary fashion. It makes it clear how important it is to inform even young children about what is happening to them and to allow them to help make decisions. Even two- or three-year-olds can decide in what order certain procedures should be carried out (for example, first the lumbar puncture to collect spinal fluid or first the bone marrow aspiration).

Fleischman and his coauthors felt it was important to emphasize that children under the age of ten can understand very well what the issues are in their case, so we must do everything we can to understand their ideas and wishes. The group was also in agreement that parents usually have to make fundamental decisions. The summary remained a bit vague in its statements about the children's involvement in the decisionmaking process, indicating that parents and caregivers must decide together to what extent they will involve the child. That isn't wrong, of course, since using a child's age as the only criterion for his or her ability to understand complex relationships is certainly not sufficient. In the end it is necessary for the members of a treatment team to be clear about the child's level of maturity.

In the section on adolescents, the working group did not go so far as to suggest treating them like adults. Instead, the approach depends on age, although they made it clear that we cannot construct a clear age scale. The participants agreed, however, that there are adolescents who are quite capable of making their own decisions. This is particularly true of those characterized by American law as "emancipated minors," which includes young people who live independently of their parents, in the military for example, or who already have a child. They did point out that the concept of the emancipated minor, which promises a young person greater freedom of choice, is continually gaining ground. They emphasized that the intention is not to minimize the family's role but that the caregivers of adolescents should respect the developing autonomy of their patients and promote their role in making decisions.

Nothing was said about potential decisions at the end of life, in other words whether and to what extent children or adolescents should have the choice of either terminating therapy completely or deciding in favor of a further experimental procedure. The article by Nitschke and collaborators (1982) that had appeared twelve years earlier is not even mentioned, which is quite remarkable. That kind of approach obviously went too far for the participants in the conference.

In 1996, M. A. McCabe and collaborators published guidelines for involving adolescents in medical decisionmaking. At the beginning they confirm that adolescents who are sick or in the terminal stage have a strong interest in being directly involved in decisionmaking, and they cite several publications (President's Commission 1983; Lantos and Miles 1989; Leikin 1989; Rushton and Lynch 1992; Evans 1995). The U.S. Patient Self-Determination Act requires that hospitals establish procedures to encourage the participation of adults in medical decisionmaking. The authors view this act as a good basis for rethinking the role of adolescents. Although most minors have no legal right to participate in decisions, the authors emphasize that instituting their right to self-determination through legislation would certainly be justifiable. The participation of adolescents occurs at three levels:

- receipt of information from the caregiver
- joint decisionmaking with parents
- autonomous decisionmaking by the adolescent, including the option of not making a decision

Adolescents were to be asked at which level they would like to be involved, although this could certainly change during the course of the illness.

According to the authors, the ability of adolescents to make decisions should be evaluated according to the three requirements for "informed consent":

- real understanding of the information
- a competent choice based on a complete understanding of risks and benefits
- absolute voluntariness without any outside pressure

The recommendations incorporate ten points that summarize the essential facts. In addition, the article includes in an appendix an instrument for identifying the level at which the adolescent wants to be involved. This paper is clearly a plea for the autonomy of adolescent patients, especially in the terminal phase of their illness.

In their article, J. P. Burns and R. D. Truog (1997) discuss ethical controversies in pediatric intensive care and the framework for children's decisionmaking. They portray the problems that arise in an intensive care unit in great detail. The authors believe that around the age of seven, children increasingly develop the ability to understand their situation and make decisions. Even if minors cannot yet decide themselves, Burns and Truog advocate fully informing the children while at the same time trying hard to find out what they are thinking. It is also important to inform a child if you are going to undertake a treatment that the child has rejected; a subterfuge is not permitted. In 2004 J. P. Burns and C. H. Rushton published a good survey article on care for dying children in the intensive care unit. In this context, it is simply a reality that children receiving artificial respiration cannot be included in the information and decisionmaking process (Burns and Rushton 2004).

The SIOP Working Committee on Psychosocial Issues in Pediatric Oncology published guidelines on how to assist a dying child in 1999 (Masera et al. 1999). In principle, the authors support including children in decisions. But in this area there is still perceptible dissension within the internationally constituted working group. Nitschke points out this deficiency in a letter to the editor (2000). Masera and Jankovic (2000), two committee members, comment on this in their response, and they also encourage other working groups to describe their experiences.

Javier R. Kane and his collaborators (2000) published a long article on supportive and palliative care for children with life-threatening illnesses and dying children. A brief section deals with decisionmaking. The task of the attending physician is to analyze the patient's situation and to present all the possibilities for the near future (including options for experimental therapies and palliative care). They point out that false hope should be equated with wishful thinking; it leads to making pointless efforts just in order to deny a painful truth. However, they do not comment at all on whether children should be involved in decisions that arise.

In the same year, Dawn E. McCallum and collaborators (2000) retrospectively analyzed the deaths of 236 children in a Canadian hospital between 1996 and 1998. Three-fourths of the children were intubated prior to their death so that in only a small percentage of cases could the question have arisen of whether or not to include them in a decision. In fact, in only one of the files was evidence found of an open discussion; in that teenager's file there was documentation that he had taken part in conversations about his care and his approaching death.

In the literature dealing with care of children in a hospice, the topic is discussed with increasing frequency. The book *Hospice Care for Children* (2001), edited by Ann Armstrong-Daily and Sarah Zarbock, can serve as an example. It includes an interesting chapter on the topic "Ethical Decision Making at the End of Life" by C. H. Rushton. First Rushton discusses collective decisionmaking by doctors and parents in substantial detail. In another section, headed "Respect for Persons," she considers the rights of children. At the beginning, she quotes the Midwest Bioethics Center Children's Rights Task Force (1995), which provided the following statement: "The ethical principle of respect for persons requires that children be recognized as individuals whose thoughts, experiences, and opinions matter, despite their developmental immaturity and legal status as minors." Rushton comments that even if children are not autonomous or self-determining, the element of respect is essential because the children's lives have a unique importance. If we want to treat children with respect, she asserts, it means recognizing and valuing who they are outside the medical context.

Rushton also assumes that severely ill children have an "accelerated" understanding of their condition and the consequences of medical treatment. In the context of decisionmaking, we should accord this knowledge an appropriate moral status. She confirms that the involvement of children and adolescents in decisionmaking varies depending on their abilities and their desire to participate. She defines four minimal requirements:

- Using appropriate concepts and depending on their stage of development, children should be informed about the nature of their condition, the proposed treatment, and the result that can be expected.
- They should know who is caring for them and performing the procedures involved in treatment.
- They should be informed about medications and treatment.
- We should find out what they are thinking and to what extent they want to be involved in decisionmaking.

Rushton clearly thinks that dying children too have a right to clear and unambiguous information and that every form of deception, lying, or concealment is an unacceptable form of paternalism. Guidelines had been established for determining the level of children's involvement in decisions about treatment (McCabe et al. 1996). She makes it clear that the child's agreement almost always requires parents' confirmation and thus as "assent" is weaker than the "consent" of the parents.

Rushton devotes a section to parents as decisionmakers and takes as her starting point the general assumption that parents act in the best interests of their child. She describes situations in which the treatment team had reasonable doubts about parental competence. This happens especially when parents have a different opinion than the medical team. Then team members often assume that parents are not able to react adequately in a crisis situation. Contrary to this assumption by professional staff, most parents are very much able to deal with the situation, and they give evidence of their responsibility as guardians by trying to find an acceptable solution for the child.

I must interject, however, that parents do not always act in their child's interest, and doctors definitely have to keep this in the back of their minds. For parents, the thought that they might lose their child is terrible. Therefore it can happen that for this very understandable reason they don't want to or can't give up the struggle against the disease. They expect their child to undergo further therapeutic measures that may prove to have many side effects and yet be ineffectual. In my opinion, the doctor must then convey to the parents that their own selfishness is causing their child to suffer unnecessarily. A lot of tact is needed to make the situation clear to parents without making them feel guilty or making them angry at the doctor who is "supposedly" accusing them of selfishness.

Finally, the author points out that parents' rights are not absolute. Children are not just members of the family, they are also members of our society. Parents' interests have a high priority, no doubt, but they should not take precedence over the child's well-being. As described above, there are rare cases when parents are not able to made a decision or to make the correct decision. Then we need to arrange for a guardian to make decisions for the child. Rushton does not comment on the difficult situation in which the child has an opinion that differs from the parents' opinion.

In the same year, an American working group reported on the results of a study in which the medical files of 146 children and adolescents who had died of cancer were evaluated (Klopfenstein et al. 2001). The goal of the study was to describe the variables that influence the care of children and adolescents at the end of life. The authors consider the question of how the determination "DNR/Do Not Resuscitate," when indicated by the treatment team, was managed in the past. They don't report at all about including the patient in the decision. In the discussion they do mention the problem briefly and support the approach that Nitschke and his collaborators described (1982). They also encourage further studies in this area in order to define the factors that influence care.

In 2003 the SIOP Working Committee on Psychosocial Issues in Pediatric Oncology published a statement on "Valid Informed Consent and Participative Decision-Making in Children with Cancer and Their Parents." The authors begin by reporting on a study from Norway that distinguished between "informed consent" and "valid informed consent" (Syse 2000). They write that "informed consent" is now often a document that a patient has legally signed without anyone actually checking and documenting what the signatory has understood. In "valid informed consent," in contrast, the emphasis is on what the patient has understood of what he or she is agreeing to and on the rational and irrational aspects of the decision. The guidelines are intended to involve this kind of consent.

The guidelines are meant to encourage doctors to inform children fully in an age-appropriate manner and to involve them in decisions. The eight points of the guidelines of the internationally constituted committee are summarized as follows:

1. The child has the right to be treated with the best medical techniques.
2. Parents are legally responsible for their children. In many countries, adolescents can make decisions independently at age eighteen; in others, earlier. The course of action must take the particular country's laws into account.
3. Children who are not legally of age do not have the right to refuse a treatment to which their parents have agreed. But they do have a right to information and should be asked for their agreement. No treatment should be undertaken without this procedure. The discussion that takes place should be documented.
4. Parents should be fully informed immediately subsequent to the diagnosis, the children as soon as possible thereafter. Communication and the exchange of information do not happen just once; they need to occur continuously. It may take several conversations before the parents or patients understand the full meaning of their situation.
5. Parents and children should be informed in detail about possible participation in a therapeutic study. This should occur in a timely manner so that there is enough time for the decision process.
6. Communication is a continuous and two-sided process. Renewed and more intensive communication is always necessary if the child has a

      recurrence, needs a more intensive treatment such as a transplant, or has entered the terminal phase.

7. Parents do not have the exclusive right to make decisions on behalf of their child. In case of doubt, if it appears that the rights of the child are not being safeguarded by the parents, the court may have to intervene. We must be aware, however, that this course of action can have negative effects on the relationship between the child and his parents.

8. Parents are often bombarded with information and must then sign declarations of consent. In many cases, they are not in a position to make competent decisions for that reason. Legal documents, however, should not serve solely as protection for doctors and institutions.

In closing, the authors of the guidelines call on doctors to treat adolescents' decisions like those of adults and to include younger children in decisions in a manner appropriate to their age. Although individual statements may be a bit vague, the basic thrust of these recommendations is unambiguous and is not adversely affected by the fact that the authors come from different countries.

In a survey article about palliative medicine in the *New England Journal of Medicine* (Himelstein et al. 2004), the topics of honesty and inclusion in decisionmaking are not discussed. They appear only in one table, where they are recommended for children over the age of six. It is remarkable that these topics are obviously not viewed as very significant. In 2005 Pamela Hinds, a nurse, and her colleagues published a study on the preferences of pediatric patients during care at the end of their lives. She had discussed this problem in earlier articles (Hinds et al. 1997, 2001; Hinds 2004). Twenty patients between the ages of ten and twenty who had a treatment-resistant cancer were interviewed seven days after they had been involved in an end-of-life decision. Three fundamentally different decisions were involved:

- enrollment in a phase-1 trial (n=7)
- adoption of a Do-Not-Resuscitate order (n=5)
- initiation of terminal care; no further treatment measures; palliative measures only (n=8)

Of the original thirty-two patients, twelve (37.5%) refused to participate in the interview because they didn't want to talk about it any more (n=5), they had no time (n=4), or they were satisfied with what they had already said and had nothing more to add (n=3). In each case, the patient, one parent, and the pediatric oncologist were interviewed separately. Eighteen patients could remember exactly what they had decided and were aware that the consequence of their decision was their death.

It would be too much to recount all the results of this study, especially since such a small group of patients was surveyed. The study does show unambiguously that adolescents are able to make important decisions for themselves, even in a life-threatening situation. Here a careful research study clearly corroborates the results of the group working with Nitschke (Nitschke et al. 1982), published more than twenty years earlier. That others would benefit from their decision was cited as an important factor by eleven of the twenty patients, an impressive finding. It was clearly important for them to participate in a phase-1 trial because other patients gain something from it, even if was harmful to themselves. This sense of responsibility for others, in the authors' opinion, may reflect the maturation effect of terminal illness on children and adolescents that earlier researchers had described. They also mention that thus far, no study in adult oncology has pointed to this kind of altruism. For adolescents, it is clear that relationships with others often play an important role in decisionmaking, and this is something doctors should take into consideration more often. Javier Kane and his collaborators (2004) had already determined that the experience of a terminal illness is a process that is dependent on relationships and that the suffering connected to it is easier to bear through close relationships with others.

In recent years a number of nurses have commented on this topic. This is a good development, since in the daily routine, nurses interact most often with the children and their parents and, in contrast to other staff, cannot withdraw during working hours. It is not easy for them to make recommendations that are aimed primarily at doctors, but they view it as important to ascertain the ideas of the children and their parents (Harrington 2005).

One study from the Netherlands that investigated which medical decisions children make in the terminal stage (Vrakking et al. 2005) should be mentioned. The authors read files and interviewed 129 doctors who had reported the death of a child between the ages of one and seventeen. The investigation centered on the children's behavior, although during a second stage sixty-three doctors were asked about how they proceeded. Forty-two of the children made fundamental decisions about how to proceed. These were:

- the decision not to treat (17 of 42)
- euthanasia (hastening death) at the express wish of the child (1 of 42)
- euthanasia at the request of the parents (no numerical data)
- euthanasia without the express wish of the parents and the child (1 of 42)
- deep sedation without artificial feeding or hydration (3 of 42)
- use of painkillers that can shorten life (21 of 42)

We are interested only in the children who were included in decisionmaking. The doctors reported that nine of seventy-six children were able to evaluate their situation correctly and make an appropriate decision. All of these children were older than ten. Seven additional children between six and eighteen were rated as at least partially competent. Twelve of the children were included in decisionmaking (including all seven of the children considered competent), two of them at their explicit request. All of the children were older than ten. It turned out that the doctors' usual approach was not to involve children under the age of twelve in making decisions. In contrast, pending decisions were discussed with all parents. In the end, the authors felt the doctors did not have a strong commitment to including the children.

In the same journal, Burns and Mitchell (2005) published a comment on this article. They note that the prevailing opinion in pediatrics is that children should participate in making decisions. They refer to the position taken by the American Academy of Pediatrics Committee on Bioethics in 1995, the gist of which is that children should be included in decisionmaking depending on their level of development. Whenever possible, they should give their assent ("assent" as a weaker form of "consent"). Unless there is a serious reason to do so, doctors should not exclude children and adolescents from decisionmaking.

Conclusion

This chapter outlined ideas about children's participation in fundamental decisions at the end of their lives as they are reflected in the literature. The topic appeared in the literature for the first time in 1977 when Nitschke and his collaborators reported on their experiences with what they called the final-stage conference. In these cases, the children and adolescents were accurately informed about their situation and told that a cure through conventional methods is no longer possible. They were presented with the possible alternative courses of action: ending all attempts at therapy or initiating an experimental therapy with a completely unclear outcome. The children were encouraged to develop their own ideas and to make a decision themselves about how to proceed. This was of course done with the agreement of the parents. In the years that followed, the authors point out repeatedly that they had good experiences with this approach and that even young children were able to make important decisions themselves.

Articles in a wide variety of publications emphasize that the children's personalities must be respected. Finally, in 2001, the Midwest Bioethics Center Children's Rights Task Force took a clear position on how to include affected children in the decisionmaking process, and they were followed by the SIOP Working Committee on Psychosocial Issues in Pediatric Oncology in 2003. The study by Hinds and collaborators (2005) basically confirmed Nitschke's results, at least in the case of adolescents. After all, the American Academy of Pediatrics was already thinking in a similar way in 1995. Our team in Tübingen also found that even very young children knew exactly how they were doing and often were able to express what they wanted clearly. Unfortunately we did not document this consistently so that we could present supporting data here. But I have no doubt about the correctness of this approach. In every case, we must consider carefully, together with the parents, why we do not want to include a child in making a decision.

Of course we can only involve children and adolescents in fundamental decisions or even leave the decisions entirely to them if we have thoroughly informed them about their situation. In fact, the increasingly positive view of including children and adolescents in decisions is simultaneously evidence that we see it as fundamentally correct to inform children fully, without keeping quiet about certain facts. This applies throughout the treatment period, not just in the terminal stage. If we handle truth this way from the very beginning, it will be easier for everyone not to diverge during the terminal phase from this approach, which is so infinitely important and helpful for everyone affected.

In a recent study (Vince and Petros 2006), the problem of young patients' autonomy, it seems to me, was taken to the extreme. The authors report on an adolescent with chronic lung disease who had to be intubated and ventilated during the terminal phase. Following an episode during which the boy was able to breathe on his own and engage in nonverbal communication, he had to be sedated and ventilated again. At that point an intensive debate developed among the team members as to whether they should allow the boy to become conscious once more in order to let him know death was approaching so that things that were pending could potentially be taken care of. The article is interesting because it discusses in depth multiple aspects of the situation related to medical ethics. This applies especially to the conflict between the team's well-intentioned paternalism and the patient's autonomy. In consultation with the parents, the team decided not to wake the patient up again, since it was possible that this would cause him substantial suffering. In closing, Vince and Petros question whether we act in the patient's best interest if we deny him the possibility of realizing his own autonomous ideas.

In a commentary on the article, Godkin (2006) notes that there had been no earlier conversation with the boy about the possibility of such a decision being required. Therefore his parents had to decide in his best interest. This means that the decision was not necessarily paternalistic. That would only have been the case if the boy had already made it clear that he wanted to be included in any decisions. Here too we see clearly the problems doctors face if they want to take patient autonomy into consideration with children and adolescents. In the final analysis, it is somewhat absurd to awaken the boy only to tell him that he is about to die. In my opinion, this would be taking our support of autonomy to the extreme, so I view this discussion as purely theoretical.

It should be emphasized in conclusion that now, a century after Freud's first comments on children's lack of knowledge, there is a general consensus that we should take patient autonomy, including the autonomy of children, seriously and respect their opinions. We must do this on a foundation of open communication from the first day of care. And because now—one hundred years after Freud—we know a lot more about the thinking of children and adolescents, we are able to support them much better when they are seriously ill than was possible for our predecessors to do. They were surely convinced they were acting in the children's best interest by not talking openly with them. It took decades of thinking intensively about this problem before a majority of pediatricians began to view understanding the "how" as the basis for the correct course of action.

I mentioned that an open and continuous dialogue with severely ill children and adolescents is a major challenge for doctors and all other members of the treatment team. Even after many years of medical practice, it is still difficult to confront a dying child or adolescent and continue the dialogue even during the final stage in the patient's life. In the interest of the children and adolescents entrusted to us, we doctors must face up to this task again and again.

References

CHAPTER ONE: Introduction

Bromberg W, Schilder P. Death and dying. A comparative study of the attitude and mental reactions toward death and dying. Psychoanal Rev 1933; 20: 133–85.

Davies DE. Talking about death with dying children (letter to the editor). N Engl J Med 2005; 352: 91.

Freud S. Totem und Tabu. Leipzig: Heller 1913.

Freud S. Die Traumdeutung. Frankfurt am Main: S. Fischer 1972, Student edition. First edition Leipzig, Vienna 1900.

Freud S. Zeitgemäßes über Krieg und Tod. In: Mitscherlich A, Richards A, Strackey J (eds). Fragen der Gesellschaft. Ursprünge der Religion. Student edition, vol. 9. Frankfurt am Main: S. Fischer 1994, 33–60. First edition Leipzig, Vienna 1915.

Guardini R. Der Tod des Sokrates. Hamburg: Rowohlt 1956.

Jens W, Küng H. Menschenwürdig Sterben. Ein Plädoyer für Selbstverantwortung. Munich: Piper 1995.

Keller G. Der Landvogt von Greifensee. In: Erzählungen: Züricher Novellen. Munich: Winkler Verlag 1972. First edition Stuttgart 1878.

Kreichbergs U, Valdimarsdóttir U, Onelov E, Henter JI, Steineck G. Talking about death with children who have severe malignant disease. N Engl J Med 2004; 351: 1175–86.

Kübler-Ross E. Interviews mit Sterbenden. Stuttgart: Kreuz-Verlag 1969.

Kübler-Ross E. On Children and Death. New York: Simon & Schuster 1985.

Lofland M. The Craft of Dying: The Modern Face of Death. Beverley Hills: Sage 1978.

Silvermann PR. Never Too Young to Know—Death in Children's Lives. New York: Oxford University Press 2000.

Tanvetyanon T. Talking about death with dying children (letter to the editor). N Engl J Med 2005: 352: 91–2.

Weisman A. On Dying and Denying: A Psychiatric Study of Terminality. New York: Behavioral Publications 1972.

Wolfe L. Should parents speak with a dying child about impending death? N Engl J Med 2004; 351: 1251–3.

Wolff G. Warum schweigen die krebskranken Kinder? Klin Padiatr 1978; 190: 287–92.

CHAPTER TWO: Children, Sickness, and Death

Freud A. Die Rolle der körperlichen Krankheit im Seelenleben des Kindes. In: Psychoanalyse für Pädagogen. Eine Einführung. Bern: Hans Huber 1971, 67–81.

CHAPTER THREE: Children in the Hospital

Bowlby J. Grief and mourning in infancy and early childhood. Psychoanal Study Child XV 1960a; 9–52.

Bowlby J. The nature of the child's tie to his mother. Int J Psychoanal 1958; 39: 350–73.

Bowlby J. Separation anxiety. Int J Psychoanal 1960b; 313–7.

Brewster AB. Chronically ill hospitalized children's concepts of their illness. Pediatrics 1982; 69: 355–62.

Bürgin D. Das Kind, die lebensbedrohliche Krankheit und der Tod. Bern: Hans Huber 1978.

Freud A, Bergmann T. Kranke Kinder. Ein psychoanalytischer Beitrag zu ihrem Verständnis. Frankfurt: S. Fischer 1972.

Freud A, Burlingham DT. War and Children. New York: International Universities Press 1943.

Gibbons MB. Psychosocial aspects of serious illness in childhood and adolescence. Curse or challenge? In: Armstrong-Dailey A, Zarbock S (eds.). Hospice Care for Children. Oxford University Press 2001, 49–67.

Kohlberg L. Development of children's orientations toward a moral order. I. Sequence in the development of moral thought. Vita Hum Int Z Lebensalterforsch 1963; 6: 11.

Petrillo M, Sanger S. Emotional Care of Hospitalized Children. Philadelphia: Lippincott 1980.

Piaget J. Sprechen und Denken des Kindes. Düsseldorf: Pädagogischer Verlag Schwann 1953.

Piaget J. Das Weltbild des Kindes. Stuttgart: Klett-Cotta 1978.

Robertson J. Some responses of young children to separation from the mothers. Nursing Times 1953; 49.

Spitz RA. Grief: A peril in infancy. New York: New York University Film Library. Ref Type: Motion Picture 1947.

Spitz RA. Vom Säugling zum Kleinkind. Stuttgart: Klett 1965.

Stern E. Kind, Krankheit und Tod. Munich: Ernst Reinhardt 1957.

CHAPTER FOUR: Children and Doctors

Freud A. Die Rolle der körperlichen Krankheit im Seelenleben des Kindes. In: Cremerius J (eds.). Psychoanalyse und Erziehungsprozess. Frankfurt am Main: S. Fischer 1971.

Freud A, Bergmann T. Kranke Kinder. Ein psychoanalytischer Beitrag zu ihrem Verständnis. Frankfurt am Main: S. Fischer 1972.

Stern E. Kind, Krankheit und Tod. Munich: Ernst Reinhardt Verlag 1957.

CHAPTER FIVE: Death and Dying in the Everyday Lives of Children

Ariès P. Geschichte des Todes. Munich: Hanser Verlag 1980.

Ariès P. Studien zur Geschichte des Todes im Abendland. Munich: Hanser Verlag 1976.

Ariès P. The Hour of Our Death. Trans. Weaver H. New York: Oxford University Press 1981. Originally published as L'Homme devant la mort. Paris 1977.

Ariès P. Western Attitudes toward Death: From the Middle Ages to the Present. Trans. Ranum PM. Baltimore: Johns Hopkins University Press 1974. Originally published as Essais sur l'histoire de la mort en Occident du Moyen Age à nos jours. Paris 1975.

Banerjee J. Through the Northern Gate: Childhood and Growing Up in British Fiction, 1719–1901. New York: Peter Lang 1996.

Bürgin D. Das Kind, die lebensbedrohliche Krankheit und der Tod. Bern: Hans Huber 1978.

Freud S. Die Traumdeutung. Frankfurt am Main: S. Fischer 1972, student edition. First edition Leipzig, Vienna 1900.

Gorer G. Death, Grief and Mourning in Contempory Britain. New York: Doubleday 1965.

Hoffmann, H (Pseudonym: Reimerich Kinderlieb). Drollige Geschichten und lustige Bilder für Kinder von 3–6 Jahren (Struwwelpeter). Frankfurt am Main: Literarische Anstalt 1845.

Joy W. Death in Puritan England. Ann Arbor: UMI Research Press 1981.

Keller G. Der Landvogt von Greifensee. In: Erzählungen: Züricher Novellen. Munich: Winkler Verlag 1972. First edition Stuttgart 1878.

Kreicbergs U, Valdimarsdottir U, Onelov E, Henter JI, Steineck G. Talking about death with children who have severe malignant disease. N Engl J Med 2004; 351: 1175–86.

Lindgren A. Die Brüder Löwenherz. Hamburg: Oetinger 1974.

Lindgren A. Mio, mein Mio. Hamburg: Oetinger 1955.

Pernick MS. Childhood death and medical ethics: an historical perspective on truth-telling in pediatrics. In: Ganos D, Lipson RE, Warren G, Weil BJ (eds.). Difficult Decisions in Medical Ethics. New York: Alan R. Liss 1983, 173–88.

Slater PG. Death and Life. Hamden, Conn.: Archon Books 1977.

Stannard D. Death in America. Philadelphia: University of Pennsylvania Press 1975.

CHAPTER SIX: Physician Paternalism versus Patient Autonomy

Binding K, Hoche A. Die Freigabe der Vernichtung lebensunwerten Lebens. Leipzig: Felix Meiner 1920.

Mitscherlich A, Mielke F. Medizin ohne Menschlichkeit. Frankfurt am Main: Fischer 1962.

Porter R. The Greatest Benefit to Mankind: A Medical History of Humanity. New York 1997.

Seidler, E. Verfolgte Kinderärzte 1933–1945. Entrechtet—geflohen—ermordet. Bonn: Bouvier 2000.

CHAPTER SEVEN: The "Precociously Mature" Child

Asperger H. Frühe seelische Vollendung bei tot-geweihten Kindern. Wien Klin Wochenschr 1969; 81: 365–6.

CHAPTER EIGHT: Healthy Children's Concepts of Death

Alexander IE, Adlerstein AM. Affective responses to the concept of death in a population of children and early adolescents. J Genet Psychol 1958; 93: 167–77.

Ames LB. Introduction: explaining death to children. In: Grollman EA (ed.). Explaining Death to Children. Boston: Beacon Press 1967, 11–5.

Anthony S. The Child's Discovery of Death. London: Routledge & Kegan Paul 1940.

Becker E. The Denial of Death. New York: Simon & Schuster 1973.

Bluebond-Langner M. The Private Worlds of Dying Children. Princeton: Princeton University Press 1978.

Bowlby J. Attachment and Loss Vol. III. Loss—Sadness and depression. New York: Basic Books 1980.

Bowlby J. Grief and mourning in infancy and early childhood. Psychoanal Study Child XV 1960b; 15: 9–52.

Bowlby J. The nature of the child's tie to his mother. Int J Psychoanal 1958; 39: 350–73.

Bowlby J. Separation anxiety. Int J Psychoanal 1960a; 41: 313–7.

Bowlby J. Robertson J, Rosenbluth D. A two-year-old goes to hospital. Psychoanal Study Child VII 1952; 82–96.

Bromberg W, Schilder P. Death and dying. A comparative study of the attitude and mental reactions toward death and dying. Psychoanal Rev 1933; 20: 133–85.

Bürgin D. Das Kind, die lebensbedrohende Krankheit und der Tod. Bern: Hans Huber 1978.

Candy-Gibbs SE, Sharp KC, Petrun CJ. The effects of age, object, and cultural/religious background on children's concepts of death. Omega 1985; 15: 329–46.

Carey S. Conceptual Change in Childhood. Cambridge, Mass.: MIT Press 1985.

Childers P, Wimmer M. The concept of death in early childhood. Child Dev 1971; 42: 1299–301.

Cotton CR, Range LM. Children's death concepts: relationship to cognitive functioning, age, experience with death, fear of death, and hopelessness. J Clin Child Psychol 1990; 19: 123–7.

Cousinet R. L'idée de la mort chez les enfants. J Psychol Normale Pathologique 1939; 36: 65–75.

Deutsch H. Absence of grief. Psa Quart 1937; 6: 12–22.

Deutsch H. A two-year-old boy's first love comes to grief. In: Jessner L, Pavenstedt E (eds.). Dynamics of Psychopathology in Childhood. New York: Grune & Stratton 1919.

Elschenbroich D. Weltwissen der Siebenjährigen. Wie Kinder die Welt entdecken können. Munich: Goldmann 2002.

Freud A. Discussion of Dr. John Bowlby's paper. Psychoanal Study Child XV 1960; 53.

Freud A, Burlingham DT. War and Children. New York: International Universities Press 1943.

Freud S. The Interpretation of Dreams. Trans. Crick J. Oxford 1999. Originally published as Die Traumdeutung. Leipzig, Vienna 1900.

Freud S. Reflections on War and Death. Trans. Brill AA, Kuttner AB. New York 1918. Originally published as Zeitgemäßes über Krieg und Tod. Vienna 1915.

Freud S. Totem und Tabu. Leipzig: Heller 1913.

Freud S. Die Traumdeutung. Frankfurt am Main: S. Fischer 1972, S. 259, student edition First edition Leipzig, Wien 1900.

Freud S. Zeitgemäßes über Krieg und Tod. In: Mitscherlich A, Richards A, Strackey J (eds.). Fragen der Gesellschaft. Ursprünge der Religion. Student edition, vol. 9. Frankfurt am Main: S. Fischer 1994, S. 33–60. First edition Leipzig, Vienna 1915.

Fulton R. On the dying of death. In: Grollman EA (ed.). Explaining Death to Children. Boston: Beacon Press 1967, 31–47.

Furman RA. Death and the young child—some preliminary considerations. In: Eissler RS, Hartman H (eds.). The Psychoanalytic Study of the Child XIX. New York: International Universities Press 1965.

Gartley W, Bernasconi M. The concepts of death in children. J Genet Psychol 1967; 110: 71–85.

Gesell A, Ilg FL. The Child from Five to Ten. New York: Harper Brothers 1941.

Grollman EA. Explaining Death to Children. Boston: Beacon Press 1967.

Grollman EA. The ritualistic and theological approach of the Jew. In: Grollman EA (ed.). Explaining Death to Children. Boston: Beacon Press 1967, p. 223–45.

Hahn A. Einstellungen zum Tod und ihre soziale Bedingtheit. Stuttgart: Ferdinand Enke 1968.

Heinicke CM. Some effects of separating two-year-old children from their parents: A comparative study. Human Relations 1956; 9: 105–76.

Hoffman SI, Strauss S. The development of children's concepts of death. Death Studies 1985; 9: 469–82.

Huang I, Lee HW. Experimental analysis of child animism. J Genet Psychol 1945; 66: 69–74.

Hug-Hellmuth H. Das Kind und seine Vorstellung vom Tode. Imago I 1912; 286–98.

Ilg FL, Bates-Ames LB. Child Behaviour. From Birth to Ten. New York: Harper & Row Publishers 1955.

Jackson EN. The theological, psychological, and philosophical dimensions of death in Protestantism. In: Grollman EA (ed.). Explaining Death to Children. Boston: Beacon Press 1967, p. 171–95.

Kane B. Children's concepts of death. J Genet Psychol 1979; 134: 141–53.

Kastenbaum R. The child's understanding of death: how does it develop? In: Grollman EA (ed.). Explaining Death to Children. Boston: Beacon Press 1967, p. 89–108.

Kastenbaum R. Aisenberg R. The Psychology of Death. New York: Springer 1972.

Kastenbaum R, Costa PT. Psychological perspectives on death. Annual Rev Psychol 1977; 28: 225–49.

Keller G. Der Landvogt von Greifensee. In: Erzählungen: Züricher Novellen. Munich: Winkler Verlag 1972. First edition Stuttgart 1878.

Klein M. A contribution to the theory of anxiety and guilt. Int J Psychoanal 1948; 29: 114–23.

Klein M. Eine Kinderentwicklung. Imago VII 1921; 251–309.

Klein M. Weaning. In: Rickman J (ed.). On the Bringing Up of Children. London: Kegan Paul 1936.

Koocher G. Childhood, death, and cognitive development. Dev Psychol 1973; 9: 363–75.

Lansdown R, Benjamin G. The development of the concept of death in children aged 5–9 years. Child Care Health Dev 1985; 11: 13–20.

Lazar A, Torney-Purta J. The development of the subconcept of death in young children: A short-term longitudinal study. Child Dev 1991; 62: 1321–33.

Lonetto R. Children's Conceptions of Death. New York: Springer 1980.

Mathews GB. Children's conception of illness and death. In: Kopelman LM, Moskop JC (eds.). Children and Health Care: Moral and Social Issues. Dordrecht: Kluwer Academic Publishers 1989, 133–46.

Maurer A. Maturation of concepts of death. Brit J Med Psychol 1966; 39: 35–41.

Mitchell ME. The Child's Attitude to Death. Chapter 6: Children's ideas about death. London: Barrie & Rockliff 1966, 55–64.

Nagera H. Children's reaction to the death of important objects: A developmental approach. Psychoanal Study Child XXV 1970; 360–401.

Nagy M. The child's theory concerning death. J Genet Psychol 1948; 78: 3–27.

Orbach I, Talmon O, Kedem P, Har-Even D. Sequential patterns of five subconcepts of human and animal death in children. J Am Acad Child Adol Psychiatr 1987; 26: 578–82.

Piaget J. Sprechen und Denken des Kindes. Düsseldorf: Pädagogischer Verlag Schwann 1953.

Piaget J. Das Weltbild des Kindes. Stuttgart: Klett-Cotta 1978.

Reilly TP, Hasazi JE, Bond LA. Children's conceptions of death and personal mortality. J Pediatr Psychol 1983; 8: 21–31.

Riley TJ. Catholic teachings, the child, and a philosophy for life and death. In: Grollman EA (ed.). Explaining Death to Children. Boston: Beacon Press 1967, 199–221.

Robertson J. Some responses of young children to separation from the mothers. Nursing Times 1953; 49.

Rochlin G. How younger children view death and themselves. In: Grollman EA (ed.). Explaining Death to Children. Boston: Beacon Press 1967, 51–73.

Rochlin G. Loss and restitution. Psychoanal Study Child VIII 1953; 288–309.

Rochlin G. The loss complex—a contribution to the etiology of depression. J Am Psychoanal Assoc 1959; 7: 299–316.

Roudinesco J, David M, Nicolas J. Responses of young children to separation from their mothers. Courrir 1952; 2: 66–78.

Safier G. A study in relationship between the life and death concepts in children. J Genet Psychol 1964; 105: 283–94.

Schilder P, Wechsler D. The attitudes of children toward death. J Genet Psychol 1934; 45: 406–51.

Selman RL, Schultz LH. Making a Friend in Youth: Developmental Theory and Pair Therapy. Chicago: University of Chicago Press 1990.

Silvermann PR. Never too Young to Know—Death in Children's Lives. New York: Oxford University Press 2000.

Solnit AJ. The dying child. Develop Med Child Neurol 1965; 7: 693–704.

Speece MW, Brent SB. Children's understanding of death: A review of three components of a death concept. Child Dev 1984; 55: 1671–86.

Stambrook M, Parker KC. The development of the concept of death in childhood: A review of the literature. Merrill-Palmer Quarterly 1987; 33: 133–57.

Stern E. Kind, Krankheit und Tod. Munich: Ernst Reinhardt 1957.

Strauss A. The animism controversy: re-examination of the Huang-Lee Data. J Genet Psychol 1951; 78: 105–11.

Sugar M. Reactions of children to divorce. Feelings and their medical significance 1972; 14: 1–4.

Sullivan HS. Personal Psychopathology, Early Formulations. New York: Norton 1972.

Tallmer M, Formanek R, Tallmer J. Factors influencing children's concepts of death. J Clin Child Psychol 1974; 3: 17–9.

Weber A. Zum Erlebnis des Todes bei Kindern. Monatsschr Psychiatr Neurol 1943; 107: 192–225.

White E, Elsom B, Prawat R. Children's conceptions of death. Child Dev 1978; 49: 307–10.

Winnicott DW. The depressive position in normal emotional development. In: Winnicott DW (ed.). Collected Papers. London: Tavistock 1954.

Wolf AWM. Helping your child to understand death. New York: Child Study Association 1973.

Wolfenstein M. How is mourning possible? Psychoanal Study Child XXI 1966; 93–123.

Yalom I. Existential Psychotherapy. New York: Basic Books 1980.

Zeligs R. Children's Experiences with Death. Springfield, Ill.: Charles C Thomas 1974.

CHAPTER NINE: Sick Children's Concepts of Death

Agranoff JH, Mauer AM. What should the child with leukemia be told? (editorial). Am J Dis Child 1965; 110: 231.

Alby N, Alby JM. L'intervention psychologique dans un centre de recherches et de traitement d'hématologie. Travail portant sur les leucémies de l'enfant. Psychiatr Enfant 1971; 14: 465–502.

Alby N, Alby JM, Chassigneux J. Aspects psychologiques de l'evolution et du traitement des leucémiques, enfants et jeune adultes, dans un centre spécialisé. Nouv Rev Franc Hématol 1967; 7: 577–88.

Alvarez W. Care of the dying. J Am Med Assoc 1952; 150: 86–91.

Asperger H. Frühe seelische Vollendung bei tot-geweihten Kindern. Wien Klin Wochenschr 1969; 81: 365–6.

Bennholdt-Thomsen C. Sterben und Tod des Kindes. Dtsch Med Wochenschr 1959; 84: 1437–42.

Bennholdt-Thomsen C. Sterben und Tod des Kindes. In: Hellbrügge T (ed.). Leben und Sterben in den Augen des Kindes. Lübeck: Hansisches Verlagskontor 1979, S. 9–27.

Bernard J, Alby JM. Problèmes psychologiques posés par la leucémie aigue de l'enfant. Courrier 1956; 6: 135–42.

Binger CM, Ablin AR, Feuerstein RC, Kushner JH, Zoger S, Mikkelsen C. Childhood leukemia: emotional impact on patient and family. N Engl J Med 1969; 280: 414–8.

Bluebond-Langner M. In the Shadow of Illness: Parents and Siblings of the Chronically Ill Child. Princeton: Princeton University Press 1996.

Bluebond-Langner M. The Private Worlds of Dying Children. Princeton: Princeton University Press 1978.

Bluebond-Langner M, DeCicco A. "Children's View of Death." In: Goldman A, Hain R, Liben S (eds.). Oxford Textbook of Palliative Care of Children. Oxford 2006.

Bluebond-Langner M, Belasco J, Goldman A. "Talking to Children about Death." Paper presented at the Yale University Institute for Social Policy Studies, 2003.

Bowlby J. Attachment and Loss Vol III, Loss—Sadness and Depression. New York: Basic Books 1980.

Braun OH. Das sterbende Kind und seine seelischen Probleme. Kinderarzt 1976; 7: 155–62.

Bürgin D. Das Kind, die lebensbedrohende Krankheit und der Tod. Bern: Hans Huber 1978.

Claflin CJ, Barbarin OA. Does "telling" less protect more? Relationships among age, information disclosure, and what children with cancer see and feel. J Pediatr Psychol 1991; 16: 169–91.

Clunies-Ross C, Lansdown R. Concepts of death, illness and isolation found in children with leukemia. Child Care Health Dev 1988; 14: 373–86.

Combs AW, Richards AC, Richards F. Perceptual Psychology: A Humanistic Approach to the Study of Persons. New York: Harper & Row 1976.

Cotton CR, Range LM. Children's death concepts: Relationship to cognitive functioning, age, experience with death, fear of death, and hopelessness. J Clin Child Psychol 1990; 19: 123–7.

Freud A, Bergmann T. Kranke Kinder. Ein psychoanalytischer Beitrag zu ihrem Verständnis. Ergebnisse aus den Wissenschaften vom Menschen. Frankfurt: S. Fischer 1969.

Glaser BG, Strauss AL. Awareness of dying. New York: Aldine Transaction 1965.

Green M. Care of the dying child. Pediatrics 1967; 40: 3–7.

Henningsen F, Ullner R. Die psychotherapeutische Betreuung sterbender und lebensbedrohlich erkrankter Kinder und ihrer Familien. In: Biermann G (ed.). Handbuch der Kinderpsychotherapie vol. 4. Munich: Ernst Reinhardt 1981, 611–23.

Hertl M. Erfahrungen mit Eltern von Leukämie-Kindern. Münch Med Wochenschr 1961; 103: 997–1002.

Hitzig WH. Psychologische Probleme bei der Behandlung der Leukämie im Kindesalter aus Standpunkt des Klinikers. Helvet Paed Acta 1965; 1: 48–55.

Inkeles A. Society, social structure, and childhood socialization. In: Clausen J (ed.). Socialization and Society. Boston: Little, Brown and Co. 1968.

Iskenius-Emmler H. Psychologische Aspekte von Tod und Trauer bei Kindern und Jugendlichen. Vol. 263. Europäische Hochschulschriften Reihe VI. Psychologie. Frankfurt am Main: Peter Lang 1988.

Jay SM, Green V, Johnson S, Caldwell S, Nitschke R. Differences in death concepts between children with cancer and physically healthy children. J Clin Child Psychol 1987; 16: 301–6.

Kane B. Children's concepts of death. J Genet Psychol 1979; 134: 141–53.

Keller G. Der Landvogt von Greifensee. In: Erzählungen: Züricher Novellen. Munich: Winkler Verlag 1972, 130. First edition Stuttgart 1878.

Kliman G. Psychological Emergencies of Childhood. New York: Grune & Stratton 1968.

Knudson AG, Natterson JM. Participation of parents in the hospital care of fatally ill children. Pediatrics 1960; 26: 482–90.

Koop CE. The seriously ill or dying child: supporting the patient and the family. Pediatr Clin North Am 1969; 16: 555–64.

Kübler-Ross E. Kinder und Tod. Zurich: Kreuz Verlag 1983.

Lansdown R, Benjamin G. The development of the concept of death in children aged 5–9 years. Child Care Health Dev 1985; 11: 13–20.

Larbig W. Zum kindlichen Todeserleben und zur Situation des todkranken Kindes im Krankenhaus. Prax Kinderpsychol Kinderpsychiatr 1974; 23: 245–55.

Morrissey JR. Children's adaption to fatal illness. Social Work 1963; 8: 81–8.

Nagy M. The child's theory concerning death. J Genet Psychol 1948; 78: 3–27.

Natterson JM, Knudson AG. Observations concerning fear of death in fatally ill children and their mothers. Psychosom Med 1960; 22: 456–65.

Nitschke R, Sexauer CL, Spencer B, Humphrey GB. Psychische Betreuung chronisch erkrankter Kinder mit progressivem Krankheitsverlauf. Mschr Kinderheilk 1985; 133: 374–8.

Nitschke R, Wunder S, Sexauer CL, Humphrey GB. The final-stage conference: The patients on research drugs in pediatric oncology. J Ped Psychol 1977; 2: 58–64.

Oehme J. Zur Klinik und Therapie akuter Leukosen des Kindes unter Beachtung physiologischer und psychologischer Besonderheiten. Med Klin 1960; 22: 956–9.

Oehme J, Janssen W, Hagitte C. Leukämie im Kindesalter. Stuttgart: Thieme 1958.

Osgood EE. Psychological factors in the care of incurable cancer. Acta Un Int Cancer 1963; 19: 5.

Plank EN. Heilpädagogik im Kinderkrankenhaus. In: Biermann G (ed.). Handbuch der Kinderpsychotherapie vol. 2. Munich: Ernst Reinhardt 1969, 989–98.

Plank EN. Hilfen für Kinder im Krankenhaus. Munich: Ernst Reinhardt 1973, 43–8.

Plank EN. Working with Children in Hospitals. Cleveland: Case Western Reserve University Press 1971.

Raimbault G. L'enfant et la mort. Des enfants malades parlent de la mort: Problèmes de la clinique du deuil. Toulouse: Edouard Privat 1975.

Raimbault G. Kinder sprechen vom Tod. Klinische Probleme der Trauer. Frankfurt: Suhrkamp 1980.

Ramachers G. Entwicklung und Bedingungen von Todeskonzepten beim Kind. Vol. 489. Europäische Hochschulschriften Reihe VI. Psychologie. Frankfurt: Peter Lang 1994.

Reilly TP, Hasazi JE, Bond LA. Children's conceptions of death and personal mortality. J Pediatr Psychol 1983; 8: 21–31.

Richmond JB, Waisman HA. Psychological aspects of management of children with malignant diseases. Am J Dis Child 1955; 89: 42–7.

Rudder de B. Über Erkenntnisschichten und Axiome heutiger Medizin. Dtsch Med Wochenschr 1950; 75: 39.

Sachtleben P. Die Betreuung des leukämiekranken Kindes und seiner Eltern. Mschr Kinderheilk 1970; 118: 14–8.

Schäfer K-H. Das Kind in Grenzsituationen des Lebens. Mschr Kinderheilk 1972; 120: 389–94.

Schowalter JE, Patterson PR, Tallmer M, Kutscher AH, Gullos SV, Peretz DE. The Child and Death. New York: Columbia University Press 1983.

Silvermann PR. Never Too Young to Know—Death in Children's Lives. New York: Oxford University Press 2000.

Speece MW, Brent SB. Children's understanding of death: a review of three components of a death concept. Child Dev 1984; 55: 1671–88.

Spinetta JJ. The dying child's awareness of death: a review. Psychol Bull 1974; 81: 256–60.

Spinetta JJ, Maloney LJ. Death anxieties in the outpatient leukemic child. Pediatrics 1975; 56: 1034–7.

Spinetta JJ, Rigler D, Karon M. Anxiety in the dying child. Pediatrics 1973; 52: 841–5.

Spranger E. Psychologie des Jugendalters. Heidelberg: Quelle & Meyer 1996.

Stern E. Kind, Krankheit und Tod. Munich: Ernst Reinhardt 1957.

Thielecke H. Theologische Ethik. 1st vol. Dogmatische, philosophische und kontrovers-theologische Grundlegung. Tübingen: Mohr 1951.

Vernick J, Karon M. Who's afraid of death on a leukemia ward? Am J Dis Child 1965; 109: 393–7.

Waechter EH. Children's awareness of fatal illness. Am J Nurs 1971; 71: 1168–72.

Waechter EH. Dying children—pattern of coping. In: Wass H, Corr CA (eds.). Childhood and Death. Washington: Hemisphere Publishing Corporation 1984. 51–68.

Wass H. Concepts of death—a developmental perspective. In: Wass H, Corr CA (eds.). Childhood and Death. Washington: Hemisphere Publishing Corporation 1984, 3–24.

Wass H, Cason L. Fears and anxieties about death. In: Wass H, Corr CA (eds.). Childhood and Death. Washington: Hemisphere Publishing Company 1984, 25–45.

Wass H, Corr CA. Childhood and Death. Washington: Hemisphere Publishing Corp. 1984.

Wolff G. Sterbebeistand bei Kindern mit onkologischen Erkrankungen. In: Hellbrügge T (ed.). Leben und Sterben in den Augen des Kindes. Lübeck: Hansisches Verlags-kontor 1979, 87–100.

Wolff G. Warum schweigen die krebskranken Kinder? Klin Padiatr 1978; 190: 287–92.

Wolff G. Was wissen denn schon die Kinder? In: Engelke E, Schmoll J-H, Wolff G (eds.). Sterbebeistand bei Kindern und Erwachsenen. Stuttgart: Ferdinand Enke 1979 49–56.

Wunnerlich A. Zur Psychologie der ausweglosen Situation. Bern: Hans Huber 1972.

Zeligs R. Children's Experiences with Death. Springfield, Ill.: Charles C Thomas 1974.

Zweig AR. Children's attitude toward death. In: Schowalter JE, Patterson PR, Tallmer M, Kutscher AH, Gullos SV, Peretz DE (eds.). The Child and Death. New York: Columbia University Press 1983.

CHAPTER TEN: Should We Tell Sick Children the Truth?

Agranoff JH, Mauer AM. What should the child with leukemia be told? (editorial). Am J Dis Child 1965; 110: 231.

Alby N, Alby JM. L'intervention psychologique dans un centre de recherches et de traitement d'hématologie. Travail portant sur les leucémies de l'enfant. Psychiatr Enfant 1971; 14: 465–502.

Alby N, Alby JM, Chassigneux J. Aspects psychologiques de l'evolution et du traitement des leucémiques, enfants et jeune adultes, dans un centre spécialisé. Nouv Rev Fr Hématol 1967; 7: 577–88.

American Academy of Pediatrics Commitee on Pediatric AIDS. Disclosure of illness status to children and adolescents with HIV infection. Pediatrics 1999; 103: 164–6.

Anderson PM. Tell the children: editorial commentary. J Clin Oncol 2000; 18: 3195.

Beale EA, Baile WF, Aaron J. Silence is not golden: Communicating with children dying from cancer. J Clin Oncol 2005; 23: 3629–31.

Bearison D. They Never Want to Tell You—Children Talk about Cancer. London: Harvard University Press 1991.

Bennholdt-Thomsen C. Sterben und Tod des Kindes. Dtsch Med Wochenschr 1959; 84: 1437–42.

Bernard J, Alby JM. Problèmes Psychologiques posés par la leucémie aigue de l'enfant. Courrier 1956; 6: 135–42.

Binger CM, Ablin AR, Feuerstein RC, Kushner JH, Zoger S, Mikkelsen C. Childhood leukemia. Emotional impact on patient and family. N Engl J Med 1969; 280: 414–8.

Bluebond-Langner M. In the Shadow of Illness: Parents and Siblings of the Chronically Ill Child. Princeton: Princeton University Press 1996.

Bluebond-Langner M. The Private Worlds of Dying Children. Princeton: Princeton University Press 1978.

Bluebond-Langner M, Belasco J, Goldman A. "Talking to Children about Death." Paper presented at the Yale University Institute for Social Policy Studies, 2003.

Bluebond-Langner M, DeCicco A. "Children's View of Death." In: Goldman A, Hain R, Liben S (eds.). Oxford Textbook of Palliative Care of Children. Oxford 2006.

Brock D. Children's competence for health care decisionmaking. In: Kopelman LM, Moskop JC (eds.). Children and Health Care: Moral and Social Issues. Dordrecht: Kluwer Academic Publisher 1989, 181–212.

Chesler MA, Barbarin OA. Childhood Cancer and the Family: Meeting the Challenge of Stress and Support. New York: Brunner & Mazel Publishers 1987.

Chesler MA, Paris J, Barbarin OA. Telling the child with cancer: Parental choices to share information with ill children. J Pediatr Psychol 1986; 11: 497–516.

Claflin CJ, Barbarin OA. Does "telling" less protect more? Relationships among age, information disclosure, and what children with cancer see and feel. J Pediatr Psychol 1991; 16: 169–91.

Collins J. Should doctors tell the truth? Harper Monthly Magazine 1927; 155: 320–6.

Davies DE. Talking about death with dying children (letter to the editor). N Engl J Med 2005; 352: 91.

Easson W. The Dying Child: The Management of the Child or Adolescent Who Is Dying. Springfield, Ill.: Charles C Thomas 1970.

Ellis R, Leventhal B. Information needs and decision-making preferences of children with cancer. Psychooncology 1993; 2: 277–84.

Evans AE, Edin S. If a child must die. N Engl J Med 1968; 278: 138–42.

Forman EN, Ladd RE. Telling the truth in the face of medical uncertainty and disagreement. Am J Pediatr Hematol Oncol 1989; 11: 463–6.

Freud A, Bergmann T. Kranke Kinder. Ein psychoanalytischer Beitrag zu ihrem Verständnis. Frankfurt am Main: S. Fischer 1972, 49.

Goldman A, Christie D. Children with cancer talk about their own death with their families. Pediatr Hematol Oncol 1993; 10: 223–31.

Graham-Pole J, Wass H, Eyberg S, Chu L, Olejnik S. Communicating with dying children and their siblings: a retrospective analysis. Death Studies 1989; 13: 465–83.

Green M. Care of the dying child. Pediatrics 1967; 40: 3–7.

Hertl M. Erfahrungen mit Eltern von Leukämie-Kindern. Münch Med Wochenschr 1961; 103: 997–1002.

Hilden J, Watterson J, Chrastek J. Tell the children. J Clin Oncol 2000; 18: 3193–5.

Hitzig WH. Psychologische Probleme bei der Behandlung der Leukämie im Kindesalter. Standpunkt des Klinikers. Helv Paediatr Acta 1965; 1: 48–55.

Hurwitz CA, Duncan J, Wolfe J. Caring for the child with cancer at the close of life. "There are people who make it, and I'm hoping I'm one of them." JAMA 2004; 292: 2141–9.

Ilg FL, Bates-Ames LB. Child Behaviour. From Birth to Ten. New York: Harper & Row 1955.

Kang T, Hoehn KS, Licht DJ, Mayer OH, Santucci G, Carroll JM, Long CM, Hill MA, Lemisch J, Rourke MT, Feudtner C. Pediatric palliative, end-of-life, and bereavement care. Pediatr Clin N Am 2005; 52: 1029–46.

Katz J. The Silent World of Doctor and Patient. New York: The Free Press 1984.

Katz, J. The Silent World of Doctor and Patient. Baltimore: Johns Hopkins University Press 2002. First edition New York 1984.

Kendrick C, Culling J, Oakhill T, Mott M. Children's understanding of their illness and its treatment within a paediatric oncology unit. Assn Child Psychol Psychiatry Newsletter 1987; 8: 16–20.

Kirkpatrick J, Hoffmann I, Futtermann EH. Dilemma of trust: Relationship between medical care givers and parents of fatally ill children. Pediatrics 1974; 54: 169–75.

Knudson AG, Natterson JM. Participation of parents in the hospital care of fatally ill children. Pediatrics 1960; 26: 482–90.

Koop CE. The seriously ill or dying child: supporting the patient and the family. Pediatr Clin North Am 1969; 16: 555–64.

Kopelman L. On the right to information and freedom of choice for the dying: is it for minors? In: Sahler OJZ (ed.). Child and Death. St. Louis: C.V. Mosby 1978, 238.

Kreicbergs U, Valdimarsdóttir U, Onelov E, Henter JI, Steineck G. Talking about death with children who have severe malignant disease. N Engl J Med 2004; 351: 1175–86.

Kreicbergs U, Valdimarsdóttir U, Steineck G. Talking about death with dying children. N Engl J Med 2005; 352: 92.

Lang P, Mitrowski C. Supportive and concrete services for teenage oncology patients. Health Soc Work 1981; 6: 42–5.

Lansky SB. Childhood leukemia. The child psychiatrist as a member of the oncology team. J Am Acad Child Psychiatry 1974; 13: 499–508.

Lansky S, Lowman JT, Vats T, Gyulay JE. School phobia in children with malignant neoplasms. Am J Dis Child 1975; 129: 42–6.

Lantos JD. Should we always tell children the truth? Perspect Biol Med 1996; 40: 78–92.

Lazarus RS. The costs and benefits of denial. In: Spinetta JJ, Deasy-Spinetta P (eds.). Living with Childhood Cancer. St. Louis: C.V. Mosby Company 1981, 50–67.

Lewis M, Otnow Lewis D. Dying children and their families. In: Schowalter JE, Patterson PR, Tallmer M, Kutscher AH, Gullos SV, Peretz DE (eds.). The Child and Death. New York: Columbia University Press 1983, 138–55.

Mack JW, Hilden JM, Watterson J, Moore C, Turner B, Grier HE, Weeks JC, Wolfe J. Parent and physician perspectives on quality of care at the end of life in children with cancer. J Clin Oncol 2005; 23: 9155–61.

Masera G, Chesler MA, Jankovic M, Ablin AR, Ben Arush MW, Breatnach F, McDowell HP, Eden T, Epelman C, Fossati B, Bellani F, Green DM, Kosmidis HV, Nesbit ME, Wandzura C, Wilbur JR, Spinetta JJ. SIOP Working Committee on psychosocial issues in pediatric oncology: guidelines for communication of the diagnosis. Med Pediatr Oncol 1997; 28: 382–5.

Masera G, Jancovic M. Care of terminal ill children with cancer (letter to the editor). Med Pediatr Oncol 2000; 34: 271–2.

Masera G, Spinetta JJ, Jankovic M, Ablin AR, D'Angio GJ, van Dongen-Melman J, Eden T, Martins AG, Mulhern RK, Oppenheim D, Topf R, Chesler MA. Guidelines for assistance to terminally ill children with cancer: a report of the SIOP Working Committee on psychosocial issues in pediatric oncology. Med Pediatr Oncol 1999; 32: 44–8.

Morrissey JR. Children's adaption to fatal illness. Soc Work 1963; 8: 81–8.

Natterson JM, Knudson AG. Observations concerning fear of death in fatally ill children and their mothers. Psychosom Med 1960; 22: 456–65.

Niethammer D. Wenn ein Kind schwer krank ist—Über den Umgang mit der Wahrheit. Berlin 2010.

Nitschke R. Regarding guidelines for assistance to terminally ill children with cancer: report of the SIOP working committee on psychosocial issues in pediatric oncology. Med Pediatr Oncol 2000; 34: 271–3.

Nitschke R, Caldwell S, Jay S. Therapeutic choices in end-stage cancer. J Pediatr 1986; 108: 330–1.

Nitschke R, Humphrey GB, Sexauer CL, Catron B, Wunder S, Jay S. Therapeutic choices made by patients with end-stage cancer. J Pediatr 1982; 101: 471–6.

Nitschke R, Meyer WH, Huszti HC. When the tumor is not the target, tell the children. J Clin Oncol 2001; 19: 595–6.

Nitschke R, Meyer WH, Sexauer CL, Parkhurst JB, Foster P, Huszti HC. Care of terminally ill children with cancer. Med Pediatr Oncol 2000; 34: 268–70.

Nitschke R, Sexauer CL, Spencer B, Humphrey GB. Psychische Betreuung chronisch erkrankter Kinder mit progressivem Krankheitsverlauf. Mschr Kinderheilk 1985; 133: 374–8.

Oehme J, Jansen W, Hagitte C. Leukämie im Kindesalter. Stuttgart: Thieme 1958.

Okamura H, Uchitomi Y, Sasako M, Eguchi K, Kakizoe T. Guidelines for telling the truth to cancer patients. Japanese National Cancer Center. Jpn J Clin Oncol 1998; 28: 1–4.

Pinkel D. Five-year follow-up of "total therapy" of childhood lymphocytic leukaemia. JAMA 1971; 216: 648–52.

Plank EN. Hilfen für Kinder im Krankenhaus. Munich: Ernst Reinhardt 1973, 43–8.

Plank EN. Leben und Tod in den Augen des Kindes. In: Hellbrügge T (ed.). Leben und Sterben in den Augen des Kindes. Lübeck: Hansisches Verlagskontor 1979, 45–77.

Purssell E. Telling children about their impending death. Br J Nurs 1994; 3: 119–20.

Raimbault G. L'enfant et la mort. Des enfants malades parlent de la mort: Problèmes de la clinique du deuil. Toulouse: Edouard Privat 1977.

Richmond JB, Waisman HA. Psychological aspects of management of children with malignant diseases. Am J Dis Child 1955; 89: 42–7.

Riehm H, Gadner H, Welte K. Die West-Berliner Studie zur Behandlung der akuten lymphoblastischen Leukämie des Kindes—Erfahrungsbericht nach 6 Jahren. Klin Pädiatr 1977; 189: 89–102.

Rudder de B. Über Erkenntnisschichten und Axiome heutiger Medizin. Dtsch Med Wochenschr 1950; 75: 39.

Sachtleben P. Die Betreuung des leukämiekranken Kindes and seiner Eltern. Mschr Kinderheilk 1970; 118: 14–8.

Sahler OJZ. Child and Death. Saint Louis: C.V. Mosby Company 1978.

Schäfer K-H. Das Kind in Grenzsituationen des Lebens. Mschr Kinderheilk 1972; 120: 389–94.

Schmeling-Kludas C. Die Arzt-Patient-Beziehung im Stationsalltag. Weinheim: Edition Medizin, VCH Verlagsgesellschaft 1988.

Schowalter JE, Patterson PR, Tallmer M, Kutscher AH, Gullos SV, Peretz D. The Child and Death. New York: Columbia University Press 1983.

Silvermann PR. Never too Young to Know—Death in Children's Lives. New York: Oxford University Press 2000.

Slavin L, O'Malley J, Koocher G, Foster D. Communication of the cancer diagnosis to pediatric patients. Impact on long-term adjustment. Am J Psychiatry 1982; 139: 179–83.

Solnit AJ. The dying child. Dev Med Child Neurol 1965; 7: 693–704.

Solnit AJ, Green M. Pediatric management of the dying child II. Child's reaction to fear of dying. In: Solnit AJ (ed.). Modern Perspectives in Child Development. Provence, N.Y.: International Universities Press 1963, 217–28.

Solnit AJ, Green M. Psychologic considerations in the management of deaths on pediatric hospital services. I. The doctor and the child's family. Pediatrics 1959; 24: 106–12.

Spinetta JJ. Communication patterns in families dealing with life-threatening illness. In: Sahler OJZ (ed.). Child and Death. St. Louis: C.V. Mosby Company 1978.

Spinetta JJ. The dying child's awareness of death: a review. Psychol Bull 1974; 81: 256–60.

Spinetta JJ, Deasy-Spinetta P. Living with Childhood Cancer. St. Louis: C.V. Mosby Company 1981.

Spinetta JJ, Deasy-Spinetta P. Talking with children who have a life-threatening illness. In: Spinetta JJ, Deasy-Spinetta P (eds.). Living with Childhood Cancer. St. Louis: C.V. Mosby Company 1981, 234.

Spinetta JJ, Maloney LJ. The child with cancer: patterns of communication and denial. J Consult Clin Psychol 1978; 46: 1540–1.

Spinetta JJ, Maloney LJ. Death anxieties in the outpatient leukemic child. Pediatrics 1975; 56: 1034–7.

Spinetta JJ, Rigler D, Karon M. Anxiety in the dying child. Pediatrics 1973; 52: 841–5.

Stern E. Kind, Krankheit und Tod. Munich: Ernst Reinhardt 1957.

Tanvetyanon T. Talking about death with dying children (letter to the editor). N Engl J Med 2005; 352: 91–2.

Tuckett AG. Truth-telling in clinical practice and the arguments for and against: a review of the literature. Nurs Ethics 2004; 11: 500–13.

Vernick J, Karon M. What should the child with leukemia be told? (letter to the editor). Am J Dis Child 1965; 110: 335.

Vernick J, Karon M. Who's afraid of death on a leukemia ward? Am J Dis Child 1965; 109: 393–7.

Waechter E. Children's awareness of fatal illness. Am J Nurs 1971; 71: 1168–72.

Waechter EH. Dying children—pattern of coping. In: Wass H, Corr CA (eds.). Childhood and Death. Washington: Hemisphere Publishing Corporation 1984, 51–68.

Wass H, Corr CA. Childhood and Death. Washington: Hemisphere Publishing Corporation 1984.

Wolfe L. Should parents speak with a dying child about impending death? N Engl J Med 2004; 351: 1251–3.

Wunnerlich A. Zur Psychologie der ausweglosen Situation. Bern: Hans Huber 1972.

Yudkin S. Children and death. Lancet 1967; 1: 37–41.

CHAPTER ELEVEN: Decisions at the End of Life

American Academy of Pediatrics. Informed consent, parental permission, and assent in pediatric practice. Pediatrics 1995; 95: 314–7.

Armstrong-Dailey A, Zarbock SF. Hospice care for children. 2d ed. Oxford: University Press 2001.

Burns JP, Mitchell C. Is there any consensus about end-of-life care in pediatrics? Arch Pediatr Adolesc Med 2005; 159: 889–91.

Burns JP, Rushton CH. End-of-life care in the pediatric intensive care unit: research review and recommendations. Crit Care Clin 2004; 20: 467–85.

Burns JP, Truog RD. Ethical controversies in pediatric critical care. New Horiz 1997; 5: 72–84.

Evans JL. Are children competent to make decisions about their own deaths? Behav Sci Law 1995; 13: 27–41.

Fleischman AR, Wolan K, Dubler NN, Epstein MF, Gerben MA, Jellinek MS, Litt IF, Miles MS, Oppenheimer S, Shaw A, van Eys J, Aughan VC. Caring for gravely ill children. Pediatrics 1994; 94: 433–9.

Godkin D. Should children's autonomy be respected by telling them of their imminent death—commentary. J Med Ethics 2006; 32: 24–5.

Harrington Jacobs H. Ethics in pediatric end-of-life care: a nursing perspective. J Pediatr Nurs 2005; 20: 360–9.

Himelstein BP, Hilden JM, Boldt AM, Weissman D. Pediatric palliative care. N Engl J Med 2004; 350: 1752–62.

Hinds PS. The hopes and wishes of adolescents with cancer and the nursing care that helps. Oncol Nurs Forum 2004; 31: 927–34.

Hinds PS, Drew D, Oakes LL, Fouladi M, Spunt SL, Church C, Furman WL. End-of-life care preferences of pediatric patients with cancer. J Clin Oncol 2005; 23: 9146–64.

Hinds PS, Oakes L, Furman W, Foppiano P, Olson MS, Quargnenti A, Gattuso J, Powell B, Srivastava DK, Jayawardene D, Sandlund JT, Strong C. Decision making by parents and healthcare professionals when considering continued care for pediatric patients with cancer. Oncol Nurs Forum 1997; 24: 1523–8.

Hinds PS, Oakes L, Furman W, Quargnenti A, Olson MS, Foppiano P, Srivastava DK. End-of-life decision making by adolescents, parents, and healthcare providers in pediatric oncology: research to evidence-based practice guidelines. Cancer Nurs 2001; 24: 122–34.

Kane JR, Barber RG, Jordan M, Tichenor KT, Camp K. Supportive/palliative care of children suffering from life-threatening and terminal illness. Am J Hosp Palliat Care 2000; 17: 165–72.

Kane JR, Hellsten MB, Goldsmith A. Human suffering: the need for relationship-based research in pediatric end-of-life care. J Pediatr Oncol Nurs 2004; 21: 180–5.

Karon M. The physician and the adolescent with cancer. Pediatr Clin North Am 1973; 20: 965–73.

Klopfenstein KJ, Hutchison C, Clark C, Young D, Ruymann FB. Variables influencing end-of-life care in children and adolescents with cancer. J Pediatr Hematol Oncol 2001; 23: 481–6.

Lantos JD, Miles SH. Autonomy in adolescent medicine: A framework for decisions about life-sustaining treatment. J Adolesc Health 1989; 10: 460–6.

Leikin SA. A proposal concerning decisions to forgo life-sustaining treatment for young people. J Pediatr 1989; 115: 17–22.

Masera G, Jancovic M. Care of terminal ill children with cancer (letter to the editor). Med Pediatr Oncol 2000; 34: 271–2.

Masera G, Spinetta JJ, Jankovic M, Ablin AR, D'Angio GJ, van Dongen-Melman J, Eden T, Martins AG, Mulhern RK, Oppenheim D, Topf R, Chesler MA. Guidelines for assistance to terminally ill children with cancer: a report of the SIOP Working Committee on psychosocial issues in pediatric oncology. Med Pediatr Oncol 1999; 32: 44–8.

McCabe MA, Rushton CH, Glover J, Murray MG, Leikin S. Implications of the patient self-determination act: Guidelines for involving adolescents in medical decision making. J Adolesc Health 1996; 19: 319–24.

McCallum DE, Byrne P, Bruera E. How children die in hospital. J Pain Symptom Manage 2000; 20: 417–23.

Midwest Bioethics Center Children's Rights Task Force. Health care treatment decision making guidelines for minors. Bioethics Forum 1995; 11: A1–16.

Niethammer D. Begleitung sterbender Kinder. In: Häberle H, Niethammer D. (eds.). Leben will ich jeden Tag. Leben mit krebskranken Kindern und Jugendlichen. Freiburg: Herder 1995, 222–9.

Niethammer D. Death of a child. In: Karim ABMF, Kuitert HM, Newling DWW, Wortman V (eds.). Death. Medical, Spiritual and Social Care of the Dying. Amsterdam: VU University Press 1998.

Niethammer D. Medizin und Unheilbarkeit bei Kindern. In: Bierich JB (ed.). Arzt und Kranker. Ethische und humanitäre Fragen in der Medizin. Tübingen: Attempto Verlag 1992, 207–24.

Niethammer D. Menschenwürdig sterben aus der Sicht des Arztes. In: Jens W, Küng H (eds.). Menschenwürdig sterben. Ein Plädoyer für Selbstverantwortung. Munich: Piper 1995.

Niethammer D. Der nichteinwilligungsfähige Patient (Proband) in der klinischen Forschung—Probleme in der Intensiv- und Notfallmedizin. In: Toellner RWU (ed.). Wissen—Handeln—Ethik. Strukturen ärztlichen Handelns und ihre ethische Relevanz. Stuttgart: Fischer 1995, 109–16.

Niethammer D. Sterbehilfe und Sterbebegleitung in der pädiatrischen Onkologie. Klin Padiatr 2003; 215: 166–70.

Niethammer D, Hoffmeister M. Die Welt der Onkologie aus der Sicht des Kinderarztes und des Psychologen. In: Braun OH (ed.). Seelsorge am kranken Kind. Stuttgart: Kreuz Verlag 1983, 66–71.

Nitschke R. Regarding guidelines for assistance to terminally ill children with cancer: report of the SIOP working committee on psychosocial issues in pediatric oncology. Med Pediatr Oncol 2000; 34: 271–3.

Nitschke R, Caldwell S, Jay S. Therapeutic choices in end-stage cancer. J Pediatr 1986; 108: 330–1.

Nitschke R, Humphrey GB, Sexauer CL, Catron B, Wunder S, Jay S. Therapeutic choices made by patients with end-stage cancer. J Pediatr 1982; 101: 471–6.

Nitschke R, Meyer WH, Sexauer CL, Parkhurst JB, Foster P, Huszti H. Care of terminally ill children with cancer. Med Pediatr Oncol 2000; 34: 268–70.

Nitschke R, Sexauer CL, Spencer B, Humphrey GB. Psychische Betreuung chronisch erkrankter Kinder mit progressivem Krankheitsverlauf. Mschr Kinderheilk 1985; 133: 374–8.

Nitschke R, Wunder S, Sexauer CL, Humphrey GB. The final-stage conference: the patient's decision on research drugs in pediatric oncology. J Pediatr Psychol 1977; 2: 58–64.

President's Commission. President's commission for the study of ethical problems in medicine and biomedical and behavioral research deciding to forgo life-sustaining treatment. Washington, D.C.: U.S. Government Printing Office 1983.

Rushton CH. Ethical decision making at the end of life. In: Armstrong-Daley A, Zarbock S (eds.). Hospice Care for Children. Oxford: University Press 2001, 323–52.

Rushton CH, Lynch ME. Dealing with advance directives for critically ill adolescents. Critical Care Nurse 1992; 12: 31–7.

Schreiber-Gollwitzer BM, Schröder HM, Niethammer D. Psychosoziale Begleitung von Kindern und Jugendlichen mit malignen Erkrankungen. Mschr Kinderheilk 2002; 150: 954–65.

Shumway C, Grossman L, Sarles R. Therapeutic Choices by Children with Cancer (letter to the editor). J Pediatr 1983; 103: 168–9.

Spinetta JJ, Masera G, Jankovic M, Oppenheim D, Martins AG, Ben Arush MW, van Dongen-Melman J, Epelman C, Medin G, Pekkanen K, Eden T. Valid informed consent and participative decision-making in children with cancer and their parents: a report of the SIOP Working Committee on psychosocial issues in pediatric oncology. Med Pediatr Oncol 2003; 40: 244–6.

Syse A. Norway: valid (as opposed to informed) consent. Lancet 2000; 356: 1347–8.

Vernick J, Karon M. Who's afraid of death on a leukemia ward? Am J Dis Child 1965; 109: 393–7.

Vince T, Petros A. Should children's autonomy be respected by telling them of their imminent death? J Med Ethics 2006; 32: 21–3.

Vrakking AM, an der Heide A, Arts WF, Pieters R, van der Voort E, Rietjens JA, Onwuteaka-Philipsen BD, van der Maas PJ, van der Wal G. Medical end-of-life decisions for children in the Netherlands. Arch Pediatr Adolesc Med 2005; 159: 802–9.

Name Index